Prescription for Disaster

The Funny Side of Falling Apart

Copyright © 2014 by Candace Lafleur

The only difference between an ordeal and an adventure is Attitude

To my twin daughters Kaitlynn and Lochlynn Labelle

May you forever embrace the funny and joyous side of life. It's kind of a family thing.

Acknowledgements

This dream of mine to write and share my experience, to make other sick people smile and laugh, never would have happened without the unwavering support of my wonderful husband, Paul Labelle. If only he would think I'm funny my life would then be complete but alas, he's too 'used' to me. Thank you to my daughters for being so cool with hospitals and my friends for hanging out at my bedside to laugh with me. And to bring brownies. Lots of brownies.

Thank you to my 'nesties' for all of your support and for being my sounding board. To Stu MacDonald for instilling a love of writing, Ron Labelle for championing me on, the NHS for all of my material and Sylvia Labelle for being my cheerleader. Thank you Tuppence Van Harn for spurring me on when I thought my dream was finished. Thank you so much to my Grandmother, Mirelle Lafleur, for her steadfast faith that I can do and overcome absolutely anything.

And thank you Sarc, for all of the adventures.

Contents

Introduction

Always look on the bright side of life....

I woke up in the rain, staring curiously up at the furious sky. The lightning had blown me clear out of the building and left me on my back in the squelching mud of the open dirt road. The storm raged above, icy raindrops pelting my face from a darkness I could barely see. I couldn't feel anything else. Just cold - my heartbeat pounding in my ears.

It was one of those moments in life when time seemed to stand still – when your thoughts race about your head with the clarity and timelessness of watching things slowly happen to someone else. I've now had many of these moments, where time stands still and all the wishing in the world won't take you back to just before life imploded to a point from which things will never quite be the same. I remember the exact date I got sick – September 20th, 2011. I remember the exact moment, though I had done nothing wrong, nothing to bring this on. I was happy and fine one moment and then my life was suddenly and irrevocably turned upside down.

It was like being hit by lightning… again.

Sound rushed back to me all at once – nearby screams of children too scared to leave the safety of the nearby building with the now shattered door. People running in the mud toward me, shouting my name. The rush of the wind and the rumble of thunder – the sound of the rain plummeting into the ground and puddles beside my

1

ears. I tried to get up, to lift my head or even my arms up to signal that I was okay but I couldn't make anything move. I remember being confused and then mentally trying to feel the outline of my body to make sure everything was still there… wait, was I missing a shoe?

Why would I be missing a shoe?

See, I've always been the type of person that things just *happen* to. I've had run-ins with terrifying wildlife like bears, mountain lions and violent overweight squirrel cartels. I've always been the type of person to fall *up* more stairs than down them and if there were ever an opportunity for things to go horribly, humiliatingly wrong it would surely happen to me. I'm an absolute magnet for disaster.

I'd been working at a summer camp in the United States teaching photography – darkroom film development, back in my adventurous late teenage years. As a Canadian I figured that I'd give working in America a go – what could possibly go wrong? I'd been teaching a group of pre-teens in the darkroom at camp – a sturdily constructed wooden shed in a clearing on the mountain. The building was raised off the ground to account for the slope of the hill and everything inside was old, donated and outdated. (what else can you expect of a darkroom at a kids' camp?) The large shed had been insulated from the inside to prevent any light from seeping in, inadvertently dulling any sound from outside and covering any windows, leaving our group without much indication as to what might be going on outside. You could be attacked by bears in that shed and you wouldn't realize it until they eventually figured out how to use the door handle.

I had gathered the class in a meadow clearing to hike together up to the darkroom – taking pictures along the way with their cameras as the rain started up. We had made a run for the darkroom shed and closed the door as the rain turned into a mild storm – giddy with relief at being out of the pouring rain and dry, ready to get on with our lesson.

The storm raged on and although we couldn't hear much of what was going on outside we could hear the wind rattling the door and the rain pelting the roof of the shed. We were ready to turn out the lights and begin, having practiced the now extinct art of arranging film into canisters in the dark. It was creepy as hell with the lights off and the door rattling, like something out of a horror movie. Perfect camp fodder as the darkness and silence of concentration was periodically pierced with anxious screams and followed by mad giggles. Having to feel our way around in the pitch black shed with the sound of rolling thunder and the trembling door was an experience in horror movie magic these kids wouldn't soon forget. Even I, as the 'mature adult' in the group kept a wary eye to the door lest a seven foot tall werewolf suddenly burst through.

Having finished the actual darkroom bit I turned the lights back on to the relief of all and reached to set the timer, an old donated metal timer with long metal hands – the only thing plugged-in throughout the entire shed aside from the light.

I gripped the long metal hand of the timer at the exact moment lightning struck the shed.

As I said, it was one of those moments when things inexplicably seem to slow down – like you are watching it happen in slow motion to somebody else. I felt the current from the hand of the timer go into my right hand through my fingers and thumb but I couldn't let go. Electricity surged through my arm and into my shoulder – incredible, hot, jolting pressure. It roared down my right side along my ribs and down to my hip where it seemed to split, rocket across my pelvis and shoot straight down both legs – blowing me off my feet and backward, out the door and into the pouring rain.

Feet splashed down around me, other counselors falling to their knees in the mud by my head. I was covered with a blanket, in the pouring rain, and told to lie still, that an ambulance was on its way. At the fear of this I found my voice and flipped out –

"Are you *nuts*?! An ambulance and hospital in *America*?! I haven't got that kind of money or insurance! I'll be fine! I'll get up in a minute – cancel the ambulance before I get charged! Is it too late to call them back? Somebody help me find my shoe!"

They paused and looked at me like I had a brain injury. The other Canadian camp counselor hovering over me told me that it was okay, the camp's insurance will take care of it because it happened at work and that we had temporary green cards – we won't be billed at all.

I looked up at her and shouted "Then what the hell is taking them so long?!"

In the end I *was* billed - $18,000 worth to be hit by lightning. Disneyland would have been much cheaper and a whole lot more fun. I called my dad the next day. Someone from the camp had already called him just after it had happened, and they told me that it would be best for me to call him directly as "his reaction was a bit strange". Apparently when they had called he first asked if I was okay, then started laughing really hard telling them that he was surprised it had taken so long for him to hear from them - this kind of stuff just happens to me regularly.

He still calls me Sparky to this day.

Incidents like these happen to me so often that nothing can really catch me by surprise anymore. I've adventured through life and was never, ever able to just do things like everyone else – though this was never my intention. My journey with illness has unsurprisingly been very much the same. From falling hospital elevators and sobbing student nurses trying to stab me, exploding chairs and being dropped off and 'lost' in a scary bit of London. Spectacular bedpan incidents and an exorcist-style stroke at the tender age of 32. These things just *happen* to me and they're just too funny to keep to myself.

It's certainly better to be laughing than to be crying, right?

Being diagnosed with a serious illness turned my world upside down – there I was, adventuring along and just waiting for the sky to open up and dump some more crazy my way when suddenly everything went still and stalled. How do you move forward with a chronic illness? How do you move forward when suddenly nothing is within your control and 'moving forward' is suddenly much more terrifying and final? We cycle through the stages of acceptance and grief – ultimately grieving lost opportunities and a life left so much unlived. I got stuck, in a dark place, for what felt like a long while. I was angry – why me? I hadn't done anything wrong. I hadn't brought this on myself. I felt depressed, hopeless. What was the point? This was going to take me and there was nothing I could do about it. My children. My husband. Would my children remember me? Would they remember my smile? Would they still be vegetarians without me? I'd left so much life unlived. I couldn't see a way out.

And then I started to laugh.

I saw my illness for what it was – an illness. It wasn't me, just a small part of me. Actually, in my case it was my suicidal immune system trying to take me out which is even *more* funny when you think about it. I looked around me and saw everything in a different light – and it was *funny*. Truly, ridiculously funny. The other patients around me had hysterical stories about side effects and hospital -gown related spontaneous public nudity. The food wasn't just terrible, it was nearly criminal. I had Bell's Palsy and was chewing toast with my hands. Hospital transport actually *lost* me and I'd become a 'doctor's pet'.

It was actually all pretty funny and I smiled to myself – I guess this was it. This was to be my next adventure.

And it was gearing up to be a wild one.

I started off 2011 as a healthy 30-year-old new mum of twins and wife to a wonderful husband who not only understood but also appreciated my unique knack for getting into trouble and injury in the most humiliating ways possible. We had laughed together through a lot over the years – incidents on airplanes, wild moose encounters and hysterical misunderstandings with social services. We'd adventured through living on three different continents and can barely get through a dinner party without bringing up a horrifying Chinese hospital story or two. He even laughed with me after I'd been hit by lightning and we have both been banned from hotels in Asia for situations that weren't quite our fault.

Being "diseased" was something that we weren't quite ready for, though. And it has completely rocked us for the last two years of our lives.

In looking back at my experience this has honestly been the funniest, craziest and in many ways the best two years I've had yet. It has also been the hardest – but I try not to dwell on that. I have had so many experiences with this illness that can only be described as "what?" that I cannot bear to let them go quietly into memory. Being pulled into secret HAZMAT bunkers and the infamous "jeans incident". A spectacular bedpan failure and the most entertaining experiences with other patients that a girl could ever ask for (which is why I now always turn down a private room as a matter of principle). The following pages contain my heart and soul over these last two years and stories so humiliating that my own mother has threatened to disown me if I published a book in my real name (which I did anyway). It is my sincere hope that you laugh with me through this illness and the crazy that comes with chronic disease, because to me laughter really is the best medicine. Well, that and some outrageously expensive drugs and doctors.

So I have this rare disease Sarcoidosis, (yeah, I had to google it too) though I often think that most days Sarcoidosis has me. Sarcoidosis is an autoimmune disease (although its status is debatable) in which your immune system basically goes bat-shit insane into a sort of hyper drive attacking a perceived threat (real or imaginary is anyone's guess). Damage/disruption of vital organ functioning is collateral damage of the scarring from chronic inflammation and the multitude of granulomas (benign tumors) which are formed by a paranoid schizophrenic immune system.

It is a rare condition that seems to be known for killing off famous American black men. Me not being famous, black, American or male the odds tell me that I shouldn't have gotten this at all – but hey. I like a challenge. I have an even rarer manifestation of Sarcoidosis – Heerfordt's Syndrome, characterized by painful zombie-eyes and the occasional bout of Bell's Palsy. Now *that's* a fun party trick, let me tell you. Sarcoidosis is brought on by having a genetic pre-disposition to autoimmune disorders combined with an environmental trigger – the exact cause is not yet known. Most cases are mild in comparison but still manage to screw up lives for anywhere from 2-5 years… or forever. (and that's about as technical as I am willing to get in this book, don't worry)

Sarc causes me to "flare", in which my joints swell and my bones feel as though they are being crushed in a vice grip. I once went to a hospital during a flare, certain that I had shattered the bones in my foot only to find through an x-ray that my bones were absolutely fine. Humiliating. A flare will also cause mind-numbing fatigue not remedied by sleep and the swelling of my lymph nodes within my lungs and throughout my system. A particularly rough flare will paralyze one side of my face and turn my eyes zombie red. It can be pretty extreme at times.

Please no, anything but hypochondria!

Anyone with a chronic illness I'm sure can understand the frustration in getting a diagnosis. I hear from people all the time that for the longest while they *knew* that something was wrong with them but they just couldn't articulate what it was.

Now, for someone like me with a horrendous fear of

being thought a hypochondriac that right there is pretty horrifying. Couple that with my over-apologetic Canadian nature and you've got a pretty entertaining patient sat in Accident and Emergency (A&E). I've been to the hospital more times than I care to count in the two and a half years since having Sarc and every time I am sure that I will be turned away and told to stop wasting their time. I refuse to go in to the hospital until my husband or work colleagues practically drag me there, and once I get there – what do I say? Every visit starts with a growly A&E receptionist barking out my name and date of birth, annoyed that I've not memorized my hospital number. I then sit quietly in the waiting room looking perfectly normal and surrounded by people gripping their stomachs, clutching bloodied bandages and yowling in torment. Oh, I'd *like* to join them in their A&E opera of despair but I know that if I let it out there is little chance I will be able to rein it back in. So I sit there quietly, wanting to scream and unsure of whether or not I will be able to stand when they call my name.

And when I finally do see the doctor, what can I say? How can I describe what is happening without sounding like a lunatic? Today, for example, I am sat in a room at A&E. I've got pink eye you see, and yes, that has put me into the hospital. Pink eye. Seriously.

However, with all of the drastic immunosuppressant's I am on (such as chemotherapy and steroids) these things cause my sarc to go haywire, flaring in waves across my body and in my brain. So I went to the A&E for pink eye. How humiliating.

Then comes actually talking to a doctor about it – once they've given you the "I cannot believe you are wasting our time with pink eye" look. I begin to stammer, my confidence faltering. They ask for my symptoms and I tell them about my goopy, red eye. My near-narcolepsy fatigue. My sarc flaring, which I suspect is from an infection of some sort. The doctor doesn't look impressed – clearly I am an idiot here for pink eye. Or maybe a drug addict. I want to stand up and shout that something is very wrong and beg them to believe me, but it is a losing battle. I am considering exit strategies and whether or not I could just sneak out and go home, pretending this never happened and that it will surely get better on its own.

Then they ask for my history and I tell them about the Sarcoidosis, the chemotherapy. The stroke. The Bell's Palsy. Their demeanor changes. Student doctors are called in to "see this". I'm popped onto a bed and IV's are going in – things suddenly become much more intense. More student nurses and offers of drugs. Specialists are on their way down as I apologize profusely for taking so much of everyone's time. I assure them that I'm certain it will go away on its own, I really am fine – to which I am usually scolded for not having come in sooner. Then I am admitted, and the real fun begins.

This is the reaction every single time, though I still have a complete, heart crushing fear of being thought a hypochondriac.

How do you explain the unexplainable? How do you explain the mind-numbing fatigue without just sounding lazy? How do you explain the fevers and chills when it is the law of nature that it never happens when you finally get to the hospital? When you want to run into the emergency room screaming "LOOK AT THIS! QUICK! SOMEBODY LOOK AT THIS BEFORE IT GOES AWAY! I need a witness!" and then by the time someone actually comes to see it (that isn't just the receptionist) the flare has subsided, damn. You are left sat in the waiting room looking like the world's biggest hypochondriac and eyeing up the exit like an Olympic sprinter.

I know it isn't just me. I know a woman with Sarc in America that frequented her local hospital like this so many times that the hospital sent her a letter asking her to stop coming to the hospital. My fear reached entirely new heights once I heard that, terrified to receive such a scathing letter from a hospital yet vowing to have it framed as art for my living room if I do.

That's what I get for not topping up my Chi

So I had gone from being totally fine to on my way out within a matter of two weeks back in the fall of 2011. I remember watching television with my husband when it suddenly felt as though someone had taken a baseball bat to my right ankle, though nothing had happened. I took off my sock to reveal a large, thin yet perfect ring of swelling around my ankle. Like a doughnut. I couldn't put any pressure on it but didn't feel it was worth bothering a doctor with as it would surely go away on its own. (only hypochondriacs go to doctors for sudden an inexplicable pain and swelling, surely.) I was doing alright for a day or so until the same thing happened to the other ankle and I resorted to crawling around the house on all fours. It was time to be seen, least of which because I couldn't even open the fridge from down there – despite having spent 2 hours fashioning a fridge opening tool comprised of a mop, a coat hanger and some pipe cleaners. It didn't work, I was never meant for engineering greatness.

At the hospital I was told that I had a kidney infection, given some antibiotics and sent on my (crawling) way home. Like a total hypochondriac. I was okay with that until both wrists did the same thing a few days later and my eyes turned red.

I had already been to the hospital and was given the bum's rush out of there – so I let my Chinese employer take care of things, arranging for me to see the preferred Chinese Traditional Medicine Doctor of the Chinese Embassy in London, at his home (very prestigious). I lived in China for a number of years before coming to London and already had a great respect for acupuncture and hot cupping (the one where you come out looking as though you've been assaulted by an octopus) so off I went with an open mind and ready for anything.

The doctor's home was typical of traditional medical doctors, deep, soft sofas and walls covered with Chinese art and diagrams of the human form. Vases of flowers dotted the room interspersed with tall glass jars filled with alcohol and decomposing snakes. I crossed my fingers that my treatment wouldn't feature these jars. (please please please please please no snake juice) I was put onto a table, poked and prodded and, as was announced to my Chinese boss, my fatness was discussed. Was I aware that I was overweight?

Yes, thank you. Very aware. Thanks.

Did I eat too much food? I don't know, probably? Exercise? Not at the moment, unless you count crawling around the house and scaling the loo like it was a small Welsh mountain. I went with "moderate".

At last, after much more rather unnecessary commentary on my physical appearance (did I dye my hair? Was I a natural blonde?) I had a diagnosis:

Low Chi.

That was it. Low Chi. Dangerously low. £500 worth of pills that I was to take four times a day that tasted like old compost kind of low chi. What did I care? I had a diagnosis that was more than "kidney infection" so I left happy with my carrier bags of pills and a syrup that tasted and looked like tar. I was good.

Until I went blind.

Yes, apparently there *is* an app for that

We are expats in the United Kingdom, here for work and part of a sub-culture of global citizens bouncing around having handed our lives over to our soulless companies for them to do with us what they wish. As such, holidays are with friends instead of family (who doesn't love a Skype Christmas!?) and we were excited to be hosting Thanksgiving for eight of our dearest American friends. They apparently don't celebrate Thanksgiving in England, a fact that occurred to me when I once asked my British flat-mate if the reason he didn't celebrate Thanksgiving was because he was Jewish.

We all have our moments.

The turkey was in the oven and everything was under way – we even had a cooking schedule on an excel spreadsheet because I am such an overachiever. I, however, was not doing so well. My eyes were blood red and I couldn't open them in the light. Peeling potatoes blind is just asking for trouble so my husband did what any husband on Thanksgiving an hour away from guest arrival would do – he drove me to the hospital and dumped me in the parking lot, rushing back home to make sure the turkey didn't dry out.

I lurched my way in to the A&E clutching an ice pack to my fallen face and a Dora the Explorer bucket to my chest (just in case this was the flu) sobbing loudly and making much more of a scene than my general sensibilities would usually allow. I was quickly put into a pitch-black room to spare my eyes and troupes of doctors padded in and out of my room – unsure of exactly what they were seeing. I had Bell's Palsy and bloody eyes with searing pain throughout my bones and joints. Had it been the beginning of April they surely would have thought I was a gag sent from an old professor. They called in everybody. Ophthalmologists. Immunologists. Pulmonologists, Virologists and Neurologists. Nobody had a clue and all of my blood tests came back normal.

Then they called in a Rheumatologist – a young doctor fresh out of med school who popped in, shined a light in my zombie like eyes and exclaimed "hold on, I've read about this somewhere" while delving onto his IPhone. I jokingly asked him if there was an "app for that" and, lo and behold it turns out that there was. Sarcoidosis, he said, which I had never heard of before. Oh, and my brain might be swelling.

It was about this time that I started to get frantic texts from my friends all having arrived for dinner at my house.

"OMG are you okay?"
"What happened? Are you coming back?"
"Turkey is awesome, by the way. "
"Natalie brought pumpkin pie."
"Do you mind if we open your Baileys?"
"Did you want us to make you a doggie bag?"
"Decide quick, it's going fast"
"Alright, Paul is bringing you some mashed potatoes and gravy."
"Never mind, just the potatoes."
"Or you could just eat there."
"Love you! Happy Thanksgiving!"

I was hungry, and desperate to get back to my hosting and friends. I didn't want to spend Thanksgiving in a dark room full of alarmist doctors. I was probably just being a hypochondriac anyway.

The hospital staff were not keen on me leaving just to pop home for dinner, even though I promised to come right back after. Not keen at all.

So I was admitted, and started a 13-day in-patient adventure in getting a definitive diagnosis full of botched lumbar punctures, broken down vehicles, falling elevators, pirate themed special needs prostitutes and a love affair with hospital macaroni and cheese suspiciously lacking in macaroni. I ended off Thanksgiving 2011 curled up with my husband in a hospital bed being spoon-fed mashed sweet potatoes and having to move my jaw up and down to chew with my hands as the right side of my face had paralyzed.

But I really can't complain – it was my most memorable Thanksgiving yet.

Prologue

So that's me, in a nutshell. I've been diseased now for three years and have now had more medical adventures than I can remember. The ones I *do* remember I've written down – and what follows is a series of adventures with family, chemo, needles, spectacular transport failures and the most entertaining ward-mates a patient could ever ask for. I've even had a stroke (and have recovered pretty well) and have just been through the absolute ringer.

The thing is, nobody shared this stuff with me when I needed it. I spent the first year of this 'adventure' feeling scared, confused and alone. I was afraid to ask questions – and even if I did I could barely understand the answer. I had checked out, resigned myself to just spectate rather than be an active participant in the whirlwind of chaos that had become my life. Everyone responded to me with sympathy or sadness. Trying to be reassuring. Saying meaningless phrases like "you'll pull through this" or "at least it's not ___". My own mother whipped out a couple of doozies like "Do you have any idea how this is effecting *me*?" All of this (okay, most) was well intended – but what I really needed was for someone to just say "Oh damn!" and then laugh with me about everything that was happening.

I've written this book to make you smile. Some of it is horrible, yes. (there may be an incident with a laxative on a train near the back) Some of it is tough to write about and most of it will make you sit back and shake your head either in horror or in laughter – hopefully a good bit of both. Each chapter holds to a theme and nothing is written in any type of chronological order – but if you've spent any time in or around a hospital you should be pretty used to randomness anyway. As you'll find I was quite ill and willing to try just about anything – praise be to dried platypus testicle elixir, if it worked even just a little bit.

So if you pick up this book and at the very least it gives

you a much needed chuckle or a reminder that things could always be worse than I am truly happy, and I thank you for sharing your journey with me too.

Now, bring on the crazy!

Chapter One: Who Doesn't Like a Good Stabbing?

Facebook:

I am happy to declare that my horrible fear of needles is now officially gone. I've just had a CT scan and was violently stabbed with a cannula line not once, but three times and I didn't cry, scream or attempt to run away.

Am hoping that my irrational fear of sharks won't be resolved in the same way.

I'll admit that before sarc I was pretty bad with needles. Like, epically bad if I'm honest. I would cry, plead, hold my breath and need someone to come with me. I would hyperventilate in the car, pace the halls of the waiting room and burst into tears when my number was called.

Up until the age of 30, yes. How embarrassing.

My husband would have to go with me (humiliating), hold my hand, tell me to look away and I would count backward, in Chinese, from 50 out loud (erm... very loud) to distract myself - my rhythmic Chinese counting getting faster and higher pitched with every second until I would near 30 and shout "Oh my god how are you not done yet take it out take it out TAKE IT OUT!!!!"Like I said, humiliating. IV's? Not happening. They'd have to gas me first.

Sarc changed all of that, though. In the last two years I have had blood tests every two weeks or more, sometimes every day or even multiple times a day. I've had countless IV's and my infamous 13 goes at a lumbar puncture (spinal tap). With each stabbing I realized that the needle was inevitable, it was going to happen whether I made a fuss or not, so why bother? Just go with it. I've since had some doozies. Crying student nurses and MRI's with contrast injections in which I swear the tech had some form of epilepsy. Blown veins and IV's gushing with blood, needles coming out and an assortment of horrors that now I don't even blink at.

But there is one thing about needles that still gets me, and that is when they *talk* about it. (who does that?!?)I was in for another round of bloods and just chilling, re-reading the Hunger Games and waiting my turn. Get called in, nice nurse, everything fine. Except my veins (of course). I took a seat in the big comfy chair, fixed my gaze on the curtain and nonchalantly told the woman to "do her worst" - and she did. Left arm, in it goes, not too bothered. But blood isn't coming out she tells me. Alright, no worries. This happens to me often, she's just going to stab me again. No problem. But she doesn't. She starts digging. I can feel it wiggling around in there as my breath catches in my throat. I make a strangled sort of noise. She tells me that she can see a bulging vein there (gag) and is just going to have to dig around a bit for it. I tell her I'm not bothered if she wants to try another one. She says she doesn't want to put me through another jab if she can help it. I assure her I don't mind (as she wiggles the needle through the flesh in my inner elbow). She counters with "I've almost got it" and pushes again. I didn't *mean* to shout, but I aggressively came out with the insistence that she try the other arm.

Bandage on and I'm breathing better - she goes for the other arm. Not a problem, I'm a total needle pro, I can handle this. And I do, very well, until blood isn't coming out of that vein either. It is not possible to will yourself to bleed. I tried. Very limited success. She then did something new: she pumped it. She *pumped my arm vein.* I could feel her fingers around the needle, matching the beats of my heart with her hand and pumping against the vein. I started to sweat. It was a cold sweat - suddenly it was just very chilly. I was sweating hard. She said she "almost" had it. My mouth got dry and I started to feel very nauseas. "Put your head back and relax" she says. Oh God, very nauseas now. The room is starting to spin and I'm breathing very quickly. The needle is still in there, moving around and she is pumping my arm and talking about blood - my blood. And then she came out with the kicker:

"I don't get why the blood isn't coming out, this is a really juicy vein"

That was it, I was out.

I came to leaned back in the chair with her and another nurse fanning me with newspapers. I was woozy and humiliated, apologizing to them profusely (I am Canadian, after all) for passing out on them. They seemed so concerned and sat me up, fanned me all over (as well as under my shirt?), gave me a drink of water and assured me that it was fine, it happens all the time (riiiiiight). After a few minutes of more excessive apologizing on my part and fanning on theirs I was deemed recovered (physically, not from shame). I stooped down to gather my things when the nurse stopped me with a concerned look on her face – I couldn't go yet -

I still hadn't given them any blood.

If you are going to make a scene make sure it's at least a good one

My biggest problem with IV's is that once they are in my arm is dead to me. God help me if they stick it in my hand, I can't even *look* at it if it is in my hand. My arm flops down to my side like a dead fish. And the thought of touching it once it is in there? Not a chance. I am convinced that any jarring of the area, despite the excessive tape, would result in a blown vein and a geyser of blood gushing out of my arm. Whether or not that is at all realistic is entirely irrelevant to me. If it moves it gushes. That is all I need to know.

This in itself creates some fun moments in hospital as really, what else is there to be doing? Showering as an in-patient with a cannula in is an adventure in itself – as not only is there a risk of dislodging the needle while dressing and undressing but I am also convinced that bad things will happen if it gets wet. Like a gremlin. So in I go spending 30 minutes preparing for a five-minute shower. I do the shuffle out of my shirt without bending my elbow. The great bra extraction and after such careful and precise removal of my upper layers I throw down my garments in triumph and glee, dancing around them in the victory and relief of not having accidentally torn the thing out of my arm. Then I shower with one arm sticking out of the shower at all times (gremlin theory) and begin the slow process of re-dressing while keeping my IV at bay *and* avoiding letting my pants touch the soapy puddles all over the floor (what is *with* ward bathrooms being wet-rooms?!)

Despite how hard I try, it just doesn't seem possible for me to have a nice, normal, uneventful moment in life. I had arrived late to the infusion clinic for my first round of chemotherapy, and was directed by a kind nurse to the last remaining lounge chair up against the window in our darkened, quiet room. The other patients were already relaxing with their tests done, IV's in and most were just kicking back, reading and offering a polite smile as I sat down and arranged my things. The overly chatty one (there's always an overly chatty one) was already off on some tangent with another patient about the horrors of the NHS and, everything as it should be, I took my place in the line outside the "blood room" for my cannula and testing.

I don't fear needles, but oh how I used to! Up until about a year and a half ago I'd flip out and sob like the poor lab tech was coming at me with a bloodied up machete. I would need someone to hold my hand and talk me through it. It would take me a good day just to prepare myself. I view it more as an inevitable this is going to happen regardless of whatever fuss I make, so what's the point in squirming? Just embrace it, let it happen and it's actually not a big deal. Unless they talk about it. Those bastards. You would think that the number one lesson they tell nurses, doctors and technicians and virtually anyone taking any kind of blood or digging around with some sort of needle – "Don't Talk About It".

My first round of chemo and I made a scene. A big, proper scene. I was sat in my little chair in the blood room, making polite small talk and determinedly looking anywhere but at the needle cart or even at the nurses themselves. There were two of them, which should have tipped me off at the start. One was a trainee. Okay, no worries. Not a big deal, I'm sure she's at least practiced on fruit before me. She has a supervisor, I'll be fine.

It wasn't fine. First she stabbed. I contained myself. Then she tried a new hole. Okay, fine. Not a big deal. My record attempts to get blood in one go is only eight. This is fine. Then she started digging. I could feel it wiggling around in there. I was still okay. Then she started talking about it. I was not okay. While digging around in the crook of my elbow she motioned to her supervisor and told him that my veins were "rolling around" and she's "having to really dig around to get one" and she "thinks she got it, but the blood isn't coming out". The supervisor commented that I was looking very pale, was I always so pale? Then came the kicker as she grumbled "yeah, I'm going to have to push this further up the vein".

My world started spinning out of control and I fell out of the chair, clinging to the bed beside me for support until I eventually hit the floor, taking with me the pile of pillows that had been stacked on the bed. The flabbergasted techs jumped back, one darting to the sink to get me some water, the other asking if I was okay.

That's when I puked on my purse.

A couple of minutes on the floor, a glass of water and a wet-wipe down later I was back in the chair and ready for another go. My only request to them? "Take blood and put the cannula in wherever you want. I'm totally fine with that. Just don't *talk* about it!"

I am coming to learn, however, that when it comes to IV's timing is everything.

The Sweater X-Ray

It never ceases to amaze me that medical professionals continue to fail to understand just how heebie-jeebie inducing cannulas are – and that even though I get that you are trying to save me an extra stabbing by just popping in a cannula "in case" when you draw blood this is actually not comforting whatsoever. Especially if I have to walk around and *do* stuff with that thing in. Why oh why would you pop a cannula into the inner part of my elbow (arm now dead to me) and *then* send me down for an x-ray of my chest? Why? Is this fun to you? Do the nurses sit around backstage and giggle at the CCTV footage afterward? (I would).

So the cannula went in, just inside my elbow – rendering my arm completely useless and my elbow unable to bend for fear of ripping out the needle and gushing blood all over the floor and walls like a scene from Carrie. I was then directed to go for a chest X-ray all the way across the hospital at the Emergency X-ray area of A&E – which was fine, it isn't like I had anything better to do and a little walk would be nice. So off I went, babying my arm as though any wrong move might cause it to fall off. I couldn't even *look* at the cannula.

I made it down to x-ray having had a pretty good time watching other people notice my arm in the elevator giving involuntary shudders and their own little heebie-jeebie attacks. People give you a wide berth when you've got those things and are wandering around freely – like they are afraid of a spraying incident as well. The radiologist led me away from the gawking crowd and to an area in the back lined with teeny tiny little yellow cubicles, each with a small bench and a door that doesn't quite reach the floor *or* the ceiling. I'll just say right here that the radiologist was a rather handsome young Australian and I wasn't the only woman in there blushing. He handed me a gown and gestured to a cubicle. I was to take everything off from the waist up, including my necklace and then wait for him to come get me for my chest x-ray. No biggie, I can do this.

But the cannula was still in. How was I to get my shirt (and necklace) off without bending my arm? My bra I could do. I've done the great bra extraction under a sweater before, easy-peasy. But I couldn't undo the strap in the back with only one hand. No matter, I would figure that out later – as I would have to figure my necklace out later as well. On to step one, getting out of this sweater.

I looked at the IV. I can *totally* do this.

I pulled on the sleeve of my immovable arm with the IV, trying to pull the sweater off in an attempt to back out of the sweater slowly and surely, until I bumped into the side of the cubicle. I didn't have a lot of space to do this and am not a small woman by any measure. Okay, change of plans, other arm first. I used my un-bendable arm to grip the sleeve of my other arm, holding it tight as I began again to back out of the sweater from the other side. It wasn't budging. I pulled harder, still not gaining much ground. Gritting my teeth and letting loose a deep, guttural growl I gave a final violent tug and slammed myself into the side of the cubicle again. Gasps were heard from the cubicles beside me as well as the seating area across the way. A woman loudly asked me if I was alright and I responded that I was totally fine, nothing to worry about! Thanks!

Clearly I was lying.

I was stood there in my jeans with one arm successfully out of my sweater and the liberated sleeve flapping around my head like a wet noodle, panting heavily from the effort. I heard the radiologist in his beautiful Aussie drawl call in the woman in the cubicle next to me- I was running out of time. I had to keep going. Still I could not bend the IV arm, but I had to get this damn thing off! How hard could it be to just take off a sweater? I made to pull it over my head in a graceful swoop when everything suddenly became very dark and very tight. I had one arm free and the other, the unbendable arm, was pinned straight up in the air, wedged between my head and the sweater that was now stuck around my chest, shoulders and face.

I tugged. I pulled. Did this sweater somehow get *smaller*?! Something was seriously wrong I realized as I grasped frantically with my one free arm at the sweater. I was trying desperately to pull it over my head to release myself from the sweater of death. I was sweating hard and panting like I was doing calisthenics in there. The radiologist returned to knock on my door, asking me if I was alright and did I need any help? I quickly bent my knees so that he couldn't see my straight unbendable arm stuck up above the space in the door and told him that I just needed a few more minutes.

I was going to die in there. There would be no turning back. The sweater would have to be cut off of my body and I would have to ride the tube home in a hospital gown top. I became frantic, reaching around behind me only to find that the sweater had become hooked on my bra strap – and that I couldn't unhook it with only one arm. Even if I could bend my IV arm and risk a CSI crime scene in an x-ray cubicle there was no way I was getting it away from my ear. I looked at the IV line to see that the tube was quickly filling with dark red blood, was it *supposed* to do that? I felt woozy now – I needed to sit down. No, I needed to get this sweater *off* of me, then I could sit down.

I pulled. I tugged. I banged into walls and turned around in circles – all with a gaping audience watching my dancing arm flailing above the cubicle door and hearing my panicked breathing grow quicker and quicker. I was like an anxiety-riddled squirrel in there – at one point I audibly pleaded with the sweater. I was sweating profusely, causing the sweater to stick to my skin and feel even more like I was being eaten by a wooly anaconda.

Alright. I had worked up enough of a sweat. The radiologist has come back and I again declined his offer of help. An X-ray isn't worth this, abort! abort! If the sweater wasn't going to come off I could at least get it back on and leave with a shred of dignity.

I slowly and painstakingly worked my arm back into the flapping sleeve of my sweater, gaining inch by inch until my wrist poked through to cool, breezy freedom with the plan of then spreading my arms and forcing the sweater back down. This plan would have worked had the thing not then caught on my necklace.

Oh, this was so, so much worse. I still had my IV arm stuck up by my ear, my head was still covered in sweater, I had one breast in the sweater and one wedged under it and now my only good arm was caught, elbow bent, also around my ear. I was stuck in every sense of the word and my cannula tube was full of my own blood. There was no turning back.

I gently leaned forward toward the door, rapped it with my elbow and managed to squeak out a humiliated and defeated "help please" to whoever was out there. A moment of silence until a gentle rap was returned on my cubicle door as a sweet voice called out "how can we help you love?"

She fetched the outstandingly hot radiologist for me and brought him to my door. My arms were stuck, they would need someone from maintenance to bring a special key to let me out, could I just sit tight? So I sat down on my little bench with my arms pinned above my head, staring at the only thing in my line of vision – the cannula full of my blood. I started to feel woozy again and called for a nurse as well.

The kind women waiting across from the cubicles chatted to me through the door, as all they could see of me were my feet and my one hand stuck up above the door. They were sweet, but I could hear the giggles. I don't even know how this kind of thing can happen, it just did. The radiologist returned with a maintenance man and a nurse and the three of them opened my door and burst into laughter, tears pouring down the hot radiologists' face as he and the nurse attempted to liberate me from my sweater. The necklace was really caught on the arm of the sweater and it was decided that the only way to get me out of it was to first remove the cannula line, but that couldn't be done in the cubicle.

31

Together they wrapped me in a gown and guided me, past the gawking waiting room, into the x-ray room so I could lay down on the table to make this easier for everybody. Warning me that she was doing this blind, the nurse reached into the depths of the sweater to remove the cannula without actually being able to see it. For a needle-phobe like me the entire concept of anyone playing with a cannula line in my arm without being able to look at what they are doing is horrifying, but I was so humiliated and desperate to get out of that hot sweater that I didn't care. I was so grateful to have that thing out that I barely noticed the blood running down my arm and dripping onto the table. I didn't care, I was nearly free. The hot radiologist and nurse unhooked my sweater from my bra and necklace and with a mighty final heave pulled it off of my head.

I lay there, half naked and panting in the gloriously cool air on the cold, hard X-ray table, freed at last from the sweater of death.

When I got back upstairs, nearly an hour later, my chemotherapy nurse asked me why my cannula had been taken out. I told her that she was bound to hear about it later and just scurried back to my chair, burying my face into my book and gearing up for a second IV to be put in again.

And when I got home I threw out that sweaty, blood soaked death-trap sweater.

Going for the hospital record – lumbar puncture fun

Life was simpler before Google, when a doctor could casually mention that they were going to do a simple procedure you hadn't before heard of and patients had to just go with it and hope for the best. They could also imagine the worst – but the very worst they could possibly imagine would still now be no match whatsoever for the worst the internet can now imagine for you via googling it. Just type in a procedure and be bombarded with photos of botch jobs, horror stories of going in for a simple bronchoscopy and coming out missing a leg. Needles getting stuck in bone and a hangnail removal resulting in a painful and drawn out death.

Well, I was in the unfortunate position of being sat in a hospital bed on day eight of captivity having just assured my team of doctors that sure, I was up for anything that could result in a diagnosis and then having frantically googled "lumbar puncture" once they had left.

Oh my god. What the internet hath shown me cannot be unseen. Needles stuck in bones. Paralysis. Bleeding into my brain. Tales of dirty needles, infection and violence. I was *terrified* to the point that my hyperventilating was heard by the nurses at their station down the hall – squeaking out an "I'm fine!" when they came to check on me. Clearly the best I could hope for was to escape death or at least get a wheelchair with streamers and a nice paint job.

In they came, not even an hour later, three of them –
ready to suck the juice out of my spine with a needle of
the size surely otherwise only used in veterinary care on
the Serengeti. Roll over, they said. It will be fine, they
said. You won't feel a thing, they said.

Like hell I wouldn't feel a thing. That needle was going
in so deep I'd probably be able to taste it. Nevertheless
I was hardly in a position to argue so I did as I was told,
exactly as I was told, and curled up into a ball of
trembling nerves, exposing my naked, curved spine
these sadistic quacks and enjoying what was certain to
be the last sensations I was to experience of having
functioning legs.

Was I ready?

"Yes... no wait!"

Yes?

"What are my chances of paralysis here?"

We explained this to you already. There are no
guarantees, but this is a simple and very common
procedure. Now touch your chin to your chest and
exhale.

"Wait!... is it okay if I wiggle my toes while you're in
there?"

What? Why?

"Just to make sure that I can. So if I wiggle my toes would that be a bad thing?"

Go ahead and wiggle your toes if you'd like. It makes no difference to us, just don't move anything else and tell us if you feel any tingling.

"Wait… what do you mean tingling? What would that mean?!"

Just that we have to make adjustments. Nothing to worry about. Alright, are you ready? We need to start.

"Yes. Sorry…. Wait! My toes feel funny."

That's because you have been wiggling them frantically and they are starting to cramp. We haven't done anything yet.

"Okay."

Are you ready now?

"Can someone hold my hand?"

In the end a nurse from the ward came to hold my hand and coach me through – and thank god she did as it was most certainly *not* a standard, common procedure. An initial sting comes from the anesthetic needle, which feels a lot like a wasp bite and then a sudden deep numbing feeling, then an intense pressure as the needle is inserted into your spine between joints and bone. I held on to that poor nurse and counted backward thinking it was surely finished when one of the doctors declared that this wasn't working, they needed a much longer needle.

Wait, what?!

This went on for some time, with the needles increasing in size until it was determined that perhaps other people should have a go. Over and over I was stung by that wasp and then wiggling my toes for dear life as long needles were pushed into my spine, only to be drawn back out with an exasperated sigh from my now team of four doctors and a crew of gasping medical students. Once someone struck bone and the needle had to be yanked out they were done – I was a lost cause and they needed a pro. There had been 11 attempts and still no success, a surgical anesthesiologist must be called in.

I was bandaged up and instructed to lay perfectly flat and pillow-less until the porters came to collect me for surgery. Oh, it's not *actual* surgery, they claimed. Just more convenient for them to do it down there where they have all of the necessary equipment in case things go wrong.

Comforting.

The porter arrived with a ward nurse, wheeling my flat white bed down the hall and to certain paralysis. Into the oversized surgical elevator we went as I saw only lights and ceiling scrolling by in my vision. The nurse was wonderfully kind and chatty, resting her arm on the metal grate of the bed as the doors closed and we started our decent to the surgical suites, chatting casually with the porter as we went.

The elevator slowed between floors, was it *meant* to do that? Apparently not given the look on the nurse's face as she gripped the side of my bed all that tighter. The elevator went dark and stopped moving – surely that wasn't meant to happen. The nurse assured me in a shaky voice that it was fine, this happens sometimes (yeah, in an abandoned Soviet hospital maybe?!?) and that we would be moving again soon – and we were, as the elevator suddenly dropped down two floors, lifting the nurse and porter off the floor and slamming them into the bed as even I caught air and landed back onto the bed like a rag-doll just in time for the elevator to rocket up three floors at what felt like warp speed – the nurse and porter (who was most definitely a large man that at that moment sounded very much like an operatic woman) screamed and clung to the rails of the bed until the elevator stopped. All was silent and still as we stood there staring at each other in disbelief, unable to comprehend what had just happened and terrified that it would happen again. The elevator started moving again, descending to the intended surgical floor with a gentle *ping* and the slow opening of the doors as though we had imagined the entire thing. The nurse and porter bolted out of the elevator, leaving me in there wild-eyed and too afraid to stand as I would surely paralyze myself as the porter reached in, one foot firmly planted outside the elevator and dragged the bed out into the hall.

We didn't say anything. We couldn't say anything. I wondered aloud if we should call somebody as we resolutely made our way down the dark hall and to the bright lights of the waiting surgical suite.

I was wheeled in, handed to the anesthesiologist and abandoned by the porter. The pale and shaken nurse handed over my notes and declared to no one that she needed to go and disappeared into the hall. The Anesthesiologist asked me if everything was alright but all I could manage was "something is seriously wrong with your elevator" as she and her team prepped me for another round of precision back-stabbing. I didn't care. A lumbar puncture was cake compared to that elevator – I wonder if they would let me take the stairs back up after?

Two more attempts and I moaned in ecstasy as the needle found its mark and my spinal fluid was drawn out bringing with it sweet relief to the intense pressure in my head. I was so joyous and relaxed that I even stopped wiggling my toes. That sweet sense of relief was so glorious that I asked them to do it again (a first for them, apparently). That feeling was worth anything just for that incredible release and I would do it again in a heartbeat.

Even after 13 attempts at a lumbar puncture and a falling elevator.

Sobbing Student Nurses with Sharp Objects

I simply cannot win when it comes to needles, and I have now accepted this. In a scenario where something could go wrong for me it most certainly will go wrong, and I will often get a new phlebotomist whose only patient before me was a grapefruit. Ces't la vie, right? Everyone has to start somewhere – why not start on me?

I had arrived at the chemo ward a little later than usual and settled into my chair, unpacking my weapons of distraction (book, laptop, iPad, chargers and fruit) and settling in for a long day. The other patients all had their cannulas in by then and, as I was on month nine of chemo at the ward, the nursing staff all were quite friendly and knew me by name.

I knew there would be a downside to being nice.

The nurses huddled together and approached me like a pack of hungry lions trying to placate a panicking, wounded gazelle. Meet Julia, they said – a new student nurse on the ward who has been shadowing the cannula nurse for the last week or so, would you mind if she did your cannula today?

What was I going to say, *no*? Why not? I replied. I'm sure she will be fine and I'm used to being stabbed. Hell, I've given enough blood over the last year to keep a vampire family of six well fed. We'll be fine. Then my eyes saw Julia.

She looked a bit shaky. Was she hyperventilating? Oh crap. This wasn't going to be good. Why was she avoiding my eye contact? Alright, alright. It will be just fine. She's got a supervisor and the other nursing staff are watching over her. Someone will jump in with a tourniquet if need be. It's fine.

Julia starts to prep her cart and wheel it over. The other nurses have backed off a bit, but they aren't leaving. A hush has fallen over the room as the other patients crane their necks to watch the show. Admittedly we don't get much for entertainment up there. She starts lifting long needles up to examine them in the light directly within my line of sight as my heebie-jeebies kick in and I shudder. "Are you alright?" a nurse inquires – I'm fine, just felt a bit of a draft. I'm fine.

The tourniquet goes on my arm and I ask her to move it up so the cannula can go in closer to my elbow. She wants to put it in my hand, as the veins there are so big and thick. *Seriously. Can we not talk about veins while doing this?!* She resigns to put it up by my elbow and starts feeling around with her fingers, finding a vein and rolling it around under her fingers. She describes it to her supervisor as I start to feel a bit nauseas, and he feels around in my arm for the same vein, rolling it around and confirming her description. I can see this is going to take a long time and that I need to get my mind off of it so I pick up my book in an attempt to distract myself. All right, she says… "sharp scratch."

It's a miss.

A complete miss. She thankfully realized it and pulled the needle out right away, her confidence faltered. The supervisor tells her it's fine, just feel for the vein again and take her time. He checks that I am alright with this and I assure him that I don't mind a bit, everyone has to start somewhere and I'm in the right place if it goes badly. She didn't like the joke and now looks visibly upset. Oh crap. I give her a smile of encouragement (*what was I thinking? Am I mental?!*) and go back to pretending to read my book. "Sharp scratch" she says.

It's another miss. What is this, Battleship?!

But she doesn't take it straight back out, she starts digging around. Oh no, this is not good. I can feel it wiggling around in there, dragging, ripping a path through my flesh. The supervisor tells her that she is nearly there. I can't look. I am starting to get really nauseas and can feel myself sweating. I want so badly to rip my arm away and throw my book at them but I don't, I keep it still and keep it together – until I heard a sob that wasn't mine. Oh my god, was she *crying*? What? I looked, I should never have looked.

The student nurse was sat there with my arm in one hand and the wiggling needle in the other, tears pouring down her face and the kindly supervisor assuring her that it was okay, she's almost got it, keep going, you're almost there. There was blood running down my arm and pooling on the blue paper towel covering her lap. My blood. This girl was sobbing and I doubt she could really even see through her tears. I was too Canadian, I assured her that she was doing a great job though the other nurses, suddenly noticing how pale and sweaty I had become ran for cups of water and papers to fan me with, calling for another nurse to set up an electric fan.

And so I sat there being stabbed repeatedly by a sobbing student nurse, fanned by two others and water being held to my lips by a fourth nurse as the cannula finally made it into a vein and the supervisor guided this poor, traumatized girl through the taping and flushing procedure – only to find that they couldn't draw blood out of the cannula. I told them they wouldn't be able to. The supervisor asked if I would mind if Julia drew blood from the other arm, assuring me that it would be much easier and quicker.

Everyone's got to learn at some point, right?

Facebook:

Took my kid in to the doctor to get her cough checked out. She was given a lollipop while I was stabbed with needles, twice. Doctor figured that she may as well get me with a couple of seasonal jabs while I was there.

I think the doctor just has a sadistic streak.

Going in Deep

Well this was a new experience for me. I arrived at my chemotherapy session all calm and ready to go, ready to wait for the usual testing in preparation for my day's infusion. Swabs were put up my nose and thrust into my groin (awkward) and I was given a very small tube for which I was meant to fill with pee.

Now, this wouldn't normally have been a problem had I not A: been on water pills and B: just polished off my second bottle of water for the morning. By the time I made it to the hospital I was near to bursting yet holding it in anticipation of that little cup. Now, thanks to high dose steroids I have what is called "cushingoid" – basically I've put on so much weight and my face and torso is so round that I now look less like an attractive young mother of two and more like Jabba the Hut in drag. Every time they give me, a now fairly large woman, a tiny bottle and point me toward a tiny bathroom expecting that I will be able to give them a sample like a normal person. What they *don't* expect is that I will emerge from the bathroom, sweating profusely covered in bits of my own urine and clutching the half full sample tube in unabashed triumph. It's like getting a pee sample from an overweight, blind epileptic. Every single time.

I finished my "sample of fun" and returned to my chair to find two nurses stood there with an ultrasound machine – surely this wasn't for me? Oh it was, I was assured. We're going for a deep vein this time, so they brought an ultrasound machine to guide the needle as it is a lot bigger than what I am used to.

Fantastic.

Oh, and this nurse is learning how to guide deep cannulas by ultrasound, so I will be describing the process to her as we go – would you mind?

Of course not, why would I mind?

Ah crap. Crap crap crap. Maybe they'll be quiet about it, it will be fine. I've passed out because of people talking about it before though, and they were just calling my veins "juicy" and giving off a little bit of description. This was going to be well and truly disgusting. I'm screwed.

So I had them take a picture of the whole thing with my phone. Because otherwise I'm not sure my husband would have believed me.

It was AWFUL. The gel went on and the tech audibly described the size and girth of my veins. They looked at the screen and discussed which vein to select, in graphic detail as well as justifying *why* they were choosing a particular one. I heard phrases like "you could slide the needle really nicely up this one" and tried to hold on to the oatmeal I'd had earlier for breakfast. We were ready, oh no wait, they had to go get a bigger needle off another cart first.

"Sharp scratch" and in it went – that sucker *felt huge*. I tried to focus on other things as the tech explained that this one is going in much deeper than what I am generally used to (why were we doing this again?!), which is why it was a bit more painful and taking a bit longer than usual. More hideous phrases like "see on the screen how we have now punctured the vein and I am sliding it in…" came out of the tech while the nurse looked on. Would I like to see the screen they asked –

hell no!

Erm.. I mean, no. Thank you. I'm good.

More twisted description from the two of them about the quality of my vein, the speed that the blood was coming out and the pressure of things that I had checked out too much to understand. This was my worst nightmare of needles.

Only a mere two years ago I was an epic screamer in these situations. I'd faint, panic, procrastinate and even lie about how many days a cannula had been in for fear of having a new one inserted. I'd gone into surgery with one needle hole and woken up with nine. I've had pools of blood from needles gone wrong on my clothes, bed, self and even other people. I'd been stabbed, poked, prodded and held on to consciousness (okay, maybe not always) through what I had thought were some pretty gross and graphic descriptions about my own veins. This, however, was the ultimate hell for a recovering needle-phobe.

There was a *reason* I never dreamed of becoming a nurse.

Chapter Two: The Stroke

I once spent an afternoon at a friend's home near Bath, England sat in a deep, flowered arm chair and enjoying a sun drenched view of the surrounding hills with my friend's 82-year-old father, comparing our strokes like they were Vietnam war stories. I don't think I had ever laughed so hard in my life, and I don't think he had either. Not that strokes are funny. But it's me. I can't even have a stroke like a normal person, and looking back on it my stroke was pretty damn funny.

The day before I hadn't really been feeling like myself, I had been flaring in my legs and hands and had been taking more painkillers than usual. Not just paracetamol, either, oh no. The "holy crap there is a unicorn dancing in the hallway" kind of painkillers. I had a strange episode where I took the kids upstairs to put them to bed and started crying at the laundry in our room that wasn't done and how the bed wasn't made. I was just so overwhelmed and called my husband to come upstairs to help me, I couldn't understand why I was crying. He couldn't either - it was very unlike me.

Looking back now, I can see how these were warning signs that something was coming, and I should have settled down and rested.

The next morning I woke up early with the kids and left my husband upstairs to sleep in a bit - I felt fine. No pain in my face, no flare pain, just my version of "normal". Sat in my comfy chair as usual and was eating a bowl of fresh fruit and soy yogurt watching cartoons with the kids (Scooby Doo is growing on me). My Chinese orange cat (we brought him over here from China and that little orange bastard has *no* appreciation) sat at the top of the stairs screeching at me (like a devil cat), angry that he was being resolutely ignored. (It's bad when your twins' first proper phrase is "shut up Dermot") I could see him out the corner of my eye but I was quite engrossed in the plight of Scooby so continued to ignore him until the poor postman arrived at the door and Dermot leapt out the window like an attack-cat determined to maul said postman to his deserving death. The postman is accustomed to our cat and managed to whack him mid-air with a package before any damage was done but his surprised screech made me swing my head far to the left in alarm – and my world immediately turned upside down.

Suddenly everything tilted and the room started spinning. I had heard people describe dizziness before like the room was spinning - but I never imagined it would be like this. It wouldn't stop and it spun and spun until it was just a blur of colors going round and round. The entire entertainment unit spun in my vision like it was a tumble dryer – I could barely make out different shapes in my own living room. I raised my left arm to my face and could just see a spinning blur of pale peach flesh mixed with the dark brown leather of my armchair. I couldn't tell which way was up, I couldn't see my children right in front of me.

I closed my eyes and clutched my head to grip the excruciating pain down the right side of my head and face - I'd never felt anything like it before, but assumed

47

it was of course some new sort of sarc flare. It felt as though the side of my face had been torn open and shocked – I couldn't feel my hands on my face, I could only feel the searing pain running down the right side of my face and neck.

I hit my head on the wall and realized that I had half flung myself out of my lazy boy chair to the right and into the wall, and I couldn't sit back up. I hung there, draped over the arm of my chair with my face mashed against the wall, clenching my eyes closed to stop the spinning – wishing just that the nausea and dizziness would stop, wishing it would all just stop.

My children were screaming and I yelled for my husband who came running down the stairs - he tells me that I was grey and violently clutching the chair, swaying to the right and then trying to correct myself. I don't remember seeing him, maybe I still had my eyes squeezed shut.

He wanted to call an ambulance, but I insisted that he and the kids just drive me to my regular hospital instead (Hammersmith, London), as surely this was just a new kind of flare and I would be able to go in and they will have my notes, I wouldn't have to start at the beginning and explain what sarcoidosis is to more hospital staff. I also didn't want to be a bother to the London ambulance service.

Neither of us knew that it was a stroke, we just thought it was a new, violent flare.

Cerebellum Strokes (as I've since found on Dr. Google) make up for only 2-6% of all strokes, so most people don't ever hear about it until they have one themselves. The strokes you see on TV and are warned about are the Cerebrum Strokes - facial droop, slurred speech, memory and cognitive impairment, etc.

Cerebellum Strokes affect your balance and motor functioning. Suddenly you cannot balance yourself and your limbs act like they have minds of their own. Neither my husband nor I had ever heard of a cerebellar stroke and we certainly didn't know the signs. We didn't know if we should call an ambulance or a priest for some sort of exorcism.

I looked like a crying, hysterical, belligerent drunk.

I couldn't balance or walk - my legs worked but I pitched so violently to the right that I couldn't stand or take a step on my own. I couldn't sit in a chair without flinging myself violently to the right and out onto the floor. Sitting in the front seat of the car I tried to touch my nose and instead whacked my husband in the face pretty hard. I just had no control. I don't remember if we talked on the way there - I just remember concentrating on breathing.

The right side of my face and neck was so, unbelievably cold. Like it had turned to ice and anything that touched it (my hand, a doctor's hand, the wind, anything) was so cold it burned. The air outside touching my face was unbearably cold but the right side of my face was also numb. I couldn't feel a touch other than just a burning cold. There was a little bit of drooping, but not enough for me to notice (the doctors told me later).

Anyway, and here is where it gets ridiculous -

So we get to the hospital and my husband drives me to the front by the emergency (no stopping zone) and I tell him to let me out here, I'll walk the couple meters to A&E and he and the kids can park and meet me in there, no biggie. He says okay and as I opened the car door and took a step toward the outside world I inadvertently launched myself out of the car face first into the back of a parked taxi. And yes, there was an audience.

There were cars behind us that couldn't get through (no stopping zone) so poor Paul ran around the car to collect me (I'd since tried to right myself - possibly looked like I was making sweet sweet love to the back of the parked taxi) and hauled me over to the side of the hospital so I could hang on to the wall and wait for him to park, get the kids out of the car (they're just 2), put them in the stroller and come get me. Poor guy.

So he drives off and I'm left standing there, clutching the exterior of the hospital for dear life and only like, maybe 30 steps away from salvation - the A&E department. I'm so close I can hear the automatic doors opening and closing from just around the corner.

So I, being an unrelenting moron, had a go at making it there on my own.

It was like one step forward - fall face first into side of building. Notice random nails sticking out of side of building (what the hell?) and try to time my next step-face launch to be big enough to avoid the next nail. Success, and I did this about five more times before a passerby came running forward to help me. I calmly explained (while crying, retching and clinging to the side of the spinning building like I'd lost all faith in gravity) that I was totally fine, my husband was just parking the car and he'll be right back - no worries.

The guy reluctantly left, to be replaced by a kind woman asking if I was in labor and needed help.

So not only was I in the midst of a severe stroke, my fatness was also being pointed out. Fantastic.

When the hospital security guy showed up (apparently a *lot* of people had reported a woman in distress outside the hospital) thankfully Paul did too. I think he gave the kids to the security guy and Paul carried me, flopping and flailing like a drunk epileptic into the hospital where the reception staff jumped up and got me a wheel chair (this turned out to not be so great, as the brakes weren't on and I continuously flung myself out of the wheelchair and onto the floor and other chairs, stroller and Paul as the wheelchair was kicked across the room. Another patient kindly put the brakes on it for me.)

Paul went to go park the car in the back (had to, damn parking wardens) and left the kids in their stroller with me in the emergency room - of course they called me first - I was the only one in the waiting room that looked as though I had been possessed by Satan himself and was doing everything but the upside down spider walk across the ceiling screaming RED RUM.

But I had the kids with me so, flailing, swaying and crying like a lunatic I asked them to please call the next person and wait until my husband returned - he should only be a minute.

He wasn't. I think he took like, 20 minutes. I literally thought I was going to die. I even called him to tell him as much. Well, I think it was him.

Somebody has a voicemail with me saying that I'm dying.

My two year old twins were brilliant - they just hung out in their stroller, gave me kisses, played with each other and told me with serious faces that I needed some medicine and maybe a glass of water. The other waiting room patients gave us a wide berth, and every one that was called before me asked the triage doctor if he was sure I couldn't go first - I declined and assured *everyone* that my husband was coming.

It became so intense that the receptionist stood in front of the double doors and watched for my husband, as soon as he saw him coming back he ran through the emergency doors and got a room ready for me - I went into triage, don't remember much aside from falling out of the chair a lot and the doctor getting annoyed that I wouldn't just "sit back and stay still". Dude, if I could do that I wouldn't be here, thanks.

We were then called in and I thankfully was able to lie down. I don't remember much from this point on, but Paul was annoyed it was going so slowly, I think everyone saw my file and assumed it was a flare so that's what they were prepping for - infection tests, pain killers, getting a room ready in rheumatology - until a third doctor came in and saw the balance issues - we explained about the facial numbness and not just pain, and he left to get on the phone to Neurology at Charing Cross hospital because some things weren't adding up for him. My pupils were going wild and I was near narcoleptic when people were trying to speak to me.

Paul had to leave (he had the kids, and the parking wardens here are *awful*) and after the doctor assured him that regardless of what happened it looked like I would be admitted, he left. I was already in much better shape than an hour ago – surely that was a good sign.

That's when things went nuts.

The doctor rushed back and somebody grabbed my arm and put a cannula in, drew blood, pumped me full of something and ran off. He told me I was being transferred, just as an ambulance crew rocked up and put me onto a stretcher. Nobody said stroke and I didn't know what was going on - but I didn't care. I was too exhausted and kept falling asleep. They gave me something in my arm for sickness and suddenly I was in an ambulance, sirens wailing and everything as I apologized profusely to the bemused ambulance staff as I didn't want to be a bother, were they sure the sirens were necessary? I remember feeling so angry as they kept me awake with a constant barrage of questions, asking me over and over my name and date of birth, where I lived and what city I was in. At one point I told them the wrong birthday and city just to be a smart ass and I was injected with something again, starting the rapid fire questioning over again as we whizzed through the streets of London with sirens blazing.

We got to Charing Cross and there was a team of about 8 doctors and nurses waiting at the door for me - still nobody said stroke. I just remember being asked to stand so they could see me walk, falling straight onto the floor and pitching to the right, then laying down on a bed with needles in both arms and people asking me questions as they ran with my bed down hallways and straight into an MRI machine.

I have no idea how or when I ended up in a hospital gown, these people are *good*.

Came out of the MRI and they were all in the hallway waiting for me - except the two specialists who were looking at the results right then. They came back a few minutes later and confirmed that I had had a severe cerebellum stroke due to a blood clot that has now passed, as I bizarrely have tears in both of the cervical arteries in my neck.

"That's it? Oh thank God. So, just a stroke? Not a flare, then? Oh thank God."

I don't think they are at all used to hearing the words "just a stroke", but laughed when they realised I have multi systemic sarcoidosis so yeah, to me this was "just a stroke".

Being the youngest person on a stroke ward by a good 40 years does have its advantages. For one, there was no shortage of conversation as my kindly ward-mates introduced themselves to me once every couple of hours and asked if I was there visiting my grandmother. One particularly delightful woman wandered around stark naked attached to machines and looking round for her cat. Another was delightfully irate with the nursing team for having re-arranged her bedroom and changed her linens to this "blue paper-like troff". For the life of her she absolutely could not find her bedside table, either. Like I said, delightful!

However, being the victim of a violent stroke at the ripe old age of 32 (I'd had a couple of TIA mini-strokes the year before) tends to make one cling to one's independence a bit more than one should having just suffered a stroke.

I was brought up in a bed from the A&E to the stroke ward with very firm instructions not to stand, drink, eat or try to hold anything. Some practitioners would be with me soon. I could speak, though not particularly well. The right side of my face had drooped somewhat, causing my speech to slur. Add that to my Canadian accent and the nurses were having a pretty hard time understanding me. And I was not, under any circumstances whatsoever, to attempt to get out of bed or stand up. If I needed to use the bathroom (I did) ring the buzzer and a nurse will come to assist me (I resolved to never pee again).

A therapist came in to assess whether or not I could have a drink of water, and when you are not allowed to drink your body knows it and sets your throat on fire. 15 minutes of demonstrating that I could suck water off a sponge stick without choking myself, then I needed a break. I didn't want a break, I just wanted the damn cup! That progressed to another agonizing 15 minutes of demonstrating the same thing, and then finally (finally!) proving that I could take tiny sips of water with her holding the cup for me. Why couldn't I just hold the cup myself??? Frustrated and needing to prove that I was not a senile invalid I reached for the cup with my right hand and flipped over the entire bedside table (those things are *not* very sturdy!) sending the jug of water, charts and those stupid sponge sticks flying across the room.

Oh. That's why.

My left arm and leg were fine, but my right arm and leg still had minds of their own with Hulk-like strength. Fascinated, I hushed the startled therapist and lifted my right arm, my eyes wide as it shot out to the side in a great sweeping arc. I had not told it to do that. I just wanted to lift it a little. Like an idiot I carefully raised my right arm up to look at my hand – the therapist watched as I punched myself in the face. As she gently starting talking about physical therapy and home help my denial faltered and I started to see this for what it was – my life had just changed. How would I brush my hair? Eat? Braid my daughters' hair? Type? *Work*?? Wait, was this permanent????

A healthcare assistant arrived with a walker (a walker?!?!) to leave by my bed so they can train me to use it over the next few days and I started hyperventilating so badly that a nurse came in and upped my meds. This was real. This wasn't funny. This was happening and I couldn't change it back. I began to cry, quietly once the nurses and therapist had left. I thought over and over again that if I could just re-live that moment and not look at the cat. If I could just not have torn my stupid brainstem in the first place. If I could just go back to 8:30am when I was sitting with my kids watching cartoons and with full control over all of my limbs. If only if only if only.

Right then. Crying about it isn't fixing anything and in all honesty this is *totally* manageable – and I had to pee. I had to pee quite badly, and there was *no way* I was going to use a bedpan, not after the great bedpan incident of 2011. Nor was I going to make some poor nurses carry me to the bathroom to watch me pee. I'm a strong, resilient 32 year old woman for god's sake – and I at least had one good arm and one good leg. There's even a stupid metal walker if I need to use it.

Alright, I can do this. I just need to break it into steps, that's all. Quick steps, as I'm close to wetting myself (which is still preferable to that bedpan idea. Cripes).

Step 1 – sit up.

Okay, this is easy peasy. The bed can do that for me. Ah yes, don't grab control with right hand- I've flung it off the bed and out of reach. Fantastic. Must remember, am now left-handed. Right arm was still swinging wildly in the air so I thought it best to just let it rest and have my left arm to all the work. My stomach muscles were useless but if I'm honest they kind of have been for a while, so I strained to push myself up with my left arm – though I was still wildly pitching to the right. I started to question whether or not this was a good idea but my bladder convinced me to keep going. I flopped over to the side of the bed, understanding for the first time just how useless and out of control my right leg really was as I tried to raise it up and did an inadvertent can-can kick high up in the air, sure I would feel the strain of that one later. No matter, the bathroom was now in sight, a mere ten or so steps away from the bed. I was sitting up, facing the right way and I had caught my breath. I was ready, my right arm hanging dead at my side and no feeling in my right leg.

Step 2 – stand

Just stand up. I've done it countless times before, just stand up. Nothing happened, I was going to have to build up some momentum first. Gripping the foot rail with my left hand I began to rock back and forth (and right), back and forth (and right, dammit) back and forth and UP AND RIGHT, staying upright only by the death grip I had on the foot rail. Why was I still pitching to the bloody right?? Oh God, the gravity and momentum had put more pressure on my bladder. This had become critical – I had to make a move.

Step 3 – walk

Yeah this was not going to happen on my own – this whole useless right leg and directional violence thing was not working out in my favor. I was going to have to use the walker – and managed to fling my right arm over to it, hook my wrist over the hand-bar and drag it over to myself while still gripping the bed for dear life, swaying around like a drunken hobo. It must have been quite a sight. I heard the familiar squeak of nursing sneakers pushing a cart down the hall and I froze like a deer in headlights, eyes wide and immobile – breathing as quietly as possible and terrified to move a muscle – surely if I was spotted trying to get up they would put a stop to my attempt and the dreaded bed pan would be brought out. Or worse, they'd carry me to the bathroom in some sort of mechanical disabled swing of shame. Like a German sex swing but with nefarious medical intentions like being lowered onto a toilet with an audience and a remote, or for bathing obese people with a hose suspended over a blow up paddling pool. I stood there frozen and alert as the nurse walked past – staying perfectly still so as not to be seen, like you're supposed to do if stalked by a velociraptor. The moment she passed my door, not even glancing my way I seized my chance and made a break for the bathroom, clinging to the walker and making a tentative step forward with my right leg.

Damn stroke. I'd forgotten how super-hero strong my right leg now was and instead of stepping forward I had can-can kicked the walker, and myself, straight ahead. The walker shot out toward the door and spun out into the hall, clanging around as it went - I fell to the floor flat on my face and splayed out like a starfish. That noise was sure to attract someone, I was nearly out of time! So I dragged myself across the floor, face down, inch by inch pulling with my left arm and pushing with my leg in a desperate army crawl toward the bathroom, so close yet so far – making it to the door only to find that my right arm was too useless to reach up and grasp the door handle.

Step 4 – humiliate self

When the nurses arrived a minute later with my dented walker they found me, lying face down on the floor by the bathroom having peed myself.

It was *still* better than risking a bedpan.

The tears in my arteries happened as a result of my medications weakening my system overall, including the arteries in my neck. About two months earlier I had had a violent coughing fit and a sudden searing pain in the back of my neck. I thought I had pulled a muscle by coughing. I even went to my doctor after a few days of no improvement, but even she figured it was a pulled muscle. These tears are very rare, even more so to have them in both arteries, and are typically caused by serious car or sporting accidents and nearly impossible to diagnose without an MRI or the like. I accepted that it was probably just a pulled muscle and let it be.

I didn't want to look like a hypochondriac, after all.

Chapter Three: Other Patients

Facebook

I had an audience during my lung function test today. Very creepy old man. Giving me the evil eye and licking his lips, mumbling something about foreigners.

It was awesome.

Private Room Hell

When I was first admitted to the hospital for Sarcoidosis nobody knew what was wrong with me. My eyes were blood red and I couldn't open them in the light, the right side of my face had paralyzed and I could barely walk or use my hands. I'd not quite realized just how seriously the hospital was taking it until I was wheeled up into the 'infectious disease' ward of Rheumatology for what was to be a very long stay. The bonus of needing to stay in the dark and possibly having an infectious disease? You get a private room – yay!

At first it was lovely. My own room. My own bathroom. There was a set of doors and a separate little corridor to get from the main hall to my room, with a hand-washing and decontamination zone for use before and after visiting my private little room. There was a television, a large window and all the privacy I wanted for visitors.

As I soon came to find out, however, my eyes couldn't

tolerate the light of the television or the window, and the curtains were permanently drawn. It was a private bat-cave of darkness and silence. Visitors were non-existent in the infectious disease ward, and the nurses offered little in the way of conversation or news of the outside world. I was in my own dark little bat-cave of despair, and the only excitement I got was trying to use the bathroom in the dark and listening to the curses of the daily cleaning staff as they reeled in shock at the result.

I was bored. Oh how I was bored. For days this went on and on. I had nothing. I couldn't read a book. I couldn't play iPad games. I couldn't even go online with my phone – I couldn't even *look* at my phone. I would sit up in bed in my dark room and watch the brightly lit hallway through my quadruple glass doors as the jubilant staff, patients and other visitors jumbled along the hallway – part of the world of being non-infectious and potentially deadly. I came to make up their conversations in my head – giving them voices and back stories vibrant and twisted enough to challenge even the most elaborate Mexican soap operas. I played music on my iPad, and cursed my husband for having merged his music with mine. The best of Norah Jones does not go well with random injections of hip-hop and gangster rap. I know, right? What the hell. Seriously.

When I started singing show-tunes to myself I figured it was possibly time for an intervention. The moment I was cleared as infectious disease free (though they still didn't know what it was) I begged to be moved to a ward (an unusual request, I gather) and vowed never,

ever to be put into a private room again.

And it was so, so worth it.

The Special Needs Pirate Prostitute Brigade

Luckily for me, every time I'm admitted to the hospital they put me onto the same Rheumatology ward, though I'm always the youngest one there by at least 35 years. The staff there know me well now and call me "the Baby". (either because of my age in comparison to the other patients on the ward or because I cry a bit when they jab me with needles. I didn't ask) I've had some fantastic roommates on that ward, oh wow.

The one to my right was a very sweet little elderly lady, 82 years old, that used to be a ballroom dancing world champion. I know this because she has Alzheimer's and introduced herself to me constantly. Constantly. She also had trouble walking, so when they gave her meds to prep her for a colonoscopy that would clean out her bowels they gave her a commode, right next to me and separated only by a rather thin curtain. The poor woman nearly blew herself off the commode a couple of times. It was extremely difficult not to giggle like a twelve year old boy at the noise and commotion coming from across the curtain. Thank God the drugs I was on removed my sense of smell.

The one across from me was even better. She was an 86 year old, loud, racist, angry Italian woman that swore at the nurses, wouldn't deal with anyone that didn't have English as a first language (and was sure to tell them why), cried that she was being abused by the food quality and slept with her pink nightdress over her head and spread eagled on her bed, buck naked with her curtains wide open. Every night.

However, the most entertaining and bizarre part of that hospital stay was definitely the rotating string of pirate-themed prostitutes with special needs, there seeing a male patient also with special needs. (go ahead and take a moment to process that). It was crazy, and for a while I wondered if I was really seeing this or if I needed to have my painkillers reduced.

Every day at around four o'clock one or two of these girls (four in total) would arrive to see their friend across the hall from me, dressed like pirate themed hookers but also clearly having special needs themselves. I saw eye patches and fishnet stockings, long head bands and red striped pinafore dresses. It was just... bizarre. They would close the curtain around his bed and you could hear them chatting (not very clearly, some due to speech impediments, some due to my lack of spy equipment that I desperately needed while in hospital (Don't send me books and flowers, I want night vision goggles and a sound gun) and laughing, but then you would hear him shout something like "Gerr off woman!" and the girls would leave in a huff.

In chatting with the nurses, I found out that they all go to a special school together and all have similar learning disabilities. She explained that their prostitute-style dress was probably just their personal style preference, but she was also confused by the pirate theme. So it wasn't just me.

The first time that the nursing staff kicked them out is when they brought in some beer and got the guy properly drunk. He tore out his IV line and went wandering down the hall talking to the walls. It was fantastically entertaining. (Hey, I'd been singing show tunes to myself at this point I was so bored, I'd take any form of entertainment I could get. I was even debating introducing *myself* to ballroom dancer, just for the conversation). Then they were kicked out and banned for, get this, *having a threesome in his cubicle.* You just can't make this stuff up. He wasn't even in a private room. He was on a shared ward with three other men and across from the room I shared with crazy one and racist two. It was fantastic.

The Prisoner Next Door

The special needs pirate nympho guy was eventually discharged and replaced with a prisoner from the jail next door to the hospital (and beside the maternity ward – what a view that was while having the twins!) – who was chained to a prison guard at all times. This was a further source of much entertainment, though the nurses insisted that they did not know what he was in jail for. There was much speculation over tea at my bedside with nurses and patients alike – the speculation growing with each day whereas he started out as maybe some sort of child support dodger and building him to be a violent necropehliac serial killer.

The worst part? Even *he* got out before I did! Paul

kindly reminded me that he wasn't going home, he was going back to group showers and prison shankings, but still. What the hell??!

What is this, a Gulag?

Every ward has a crazy on it. Same as they will always have a Silent Sulker, a Chatty McChatterson and a person with poor hearing and the most unbelievably loud mobile phone ringtone. Such is the way of the world.

The crazy this week took the form of an angry middle aged Russian woman sat directly across from me and in perfect view. Oh how I was looking forward to the days' antics once I'd realized just how good this was going to get. Brilliantly enough she was also the person with poor hearing and the most unbelievably loud mobile phone ringtone – all to Britney Spears songs. Amazing. The nurses *hated* this woman, obvious despite their painstaking attempts to remain professional. The health care assistants hated this woman, as did the cleaning staff, catering staff and even other patients.

I couldn't have asked for more.

Apparently she had been coming for a week of infusions and was on her last day. She didn't show up for the first two days and was hours late for the remaining three, despite staying in a hotel across from the hospital (which was *not* to her standards) and furious that because of this things went so slowly and continuously ruined her evening plans. The nurses explained to her, over and over that had she arrived on time things would have gone smoothly but this woman was more about talking than listening. This woman could not leave anything alone and just wanted to complain, about everything and anything. Any time a nurse passed she would shout "Hallo, hallo, hallo, hallo... HALLO!" until the nurse took a deep calming breath and went over to see what she needed. She never needed anything, just wanted to complain about the horrid treatment she was receiving and how dare that nurse ignore her. She shouldn't have to shout herself hoarse to get her attention! The nurse would repeat that she needed to complain to the hospital complaints and patient liaison unit and make her escape – leaving the Russian to shout about being ignored and mistreated.

Another nurse would come by, hurrying her steps as she darted past the Russian to get to the other patients, feigning deafness to the Russian's shouts of "Hallo, hallo, hallo, HALLO." She figured out that if she presses the call button a nurse *has* to appear – though they were adamant with her that it was a help button and not a complaint button after the first 10 minutes of her frantic button mashing.

Lunch arrived via an exhausted looking woman with a loaded cart, doing her best to hand out our pre-ordered meals and get on her way. Oh God, the Russian got the wrong meal.

"I ordered ze SCHNITZEL! NOT ZE RATATOUILLE! Why you treat me like peasant piece of shit!? I look like peasant? I look like your rubbish? I ordered ze SCHNITZEL! BRING ME ZE SCHNITZEL!" and then she *threw* the ratatouille onto the floor at the feet of the poor lunch woman – who stammered and tried to explain that she had ordered the schnitzel, but for dinner not lunch. A nurse heard the commotion and came to the lunch lady's rescue – explaining again to the Russian that she had ordered the ratatouille for lunch and that the kitchen was now closed, she couldn't order anything else. As she had thrown her lunch on the floor she would now have to go downstairs to buy something that she wanted for lunch, or they could give her a piece of fruit and a sandwich. Well the Russian then lost her mind, shouting and swearing that they were starving her and she was losing weight and they cannot treat sick people this way – oh, it was a rant of epic proportions. The lunch lady left to deliver the cold remains of lunch to the other patients as the nursing staff again explained to the Russian about the hospital's complaints procedure.

This went on for hours – the Russian calling out "Hallo, Hallo, why are you ignoring me?!" to every single person that came within sight of her chair. Other patients pretended to sleep to avoid her barrage of complaints. They put on headphones to tune her out. The nurses couldn't, they were stuck with this woman, and began using phrases like "We have many things to do and it is my turn to talk, your turn to listen" as I giggled at the absurdity of it all and yet wanted to applaud the staff for all they were putting up with. Everyone that passed by was pestered by this woman for something – scissors, fill her water cup (that was in reach), to complain to…. Another patient walked past and the Russian pestered her to get a nurse to come to her – the patient rounded on her, telling the Russian that she should be ashamed of herself for how awful and rude she has been to every person in here. The Russian shot to her feet (quite spry for being so feeble) and unleashed a barrage of abuse and profanities, my favorite being that the woman was an "uneducated peasant scum". The rest of us were sat up in our chairs, alert and attentive – halfway to forming a circle around them with our IV poles and chanting "Fight! Fight! Fight!"

In my 11 months of chemotherapy I have never before seen such celebration when a patient left for the day. Cheers erupted before she was even out of earshot. Chocolates were passed around and the nursing staff were warmly and lovingly applauded. That woman was properly crazy and oh, how I will miss her.

And if that's not a magical Christmas moment I don't know what is.

Facebook

Day 13 of Captivity: I just asked my team of doctors if I would be going home any time soon or if I should go ahead and tell my husband to start dating other people.

Patsy – the secret to quick, unsustainable weight loss

The doctors began to notice that my meal trays were

returning to the kitchen relatively untouched – to the point that my meals started to arrive on bright red trays that were weighed after I handed them back. I needed to eat, they said – to build up strength and recovery, they said. But I couldn't eat.

Not with the most disgusting ward-mate of all time sat across from me on the ward.

Patsy was a vibrant middle-aged Irish woman. She was also loud, blunt, terribly racist and had very little control over her many bodily functions. Patsy would burp, fart, moan, groan, rumble, puke and crap herself – usually only around meal times. I suspect this was because she would be woken up for meals and her body would get going – forcing the rest of us to wolf down as much as we could of our meals before Patsy tried to sit up and really got going – at which point we'd all be staring woefully at the remains of our lunchtime curry and turning various shades of green as we tried to hold it down.

Facebook

2:46
Patsy: "Somebody get the nice black nurse and tell her I shat myself again"

3:37
When Patsy poops in the bedpan she congratulates herself and makes the nurse comment on the size.

3:51

Patsy has a mobile phone with the loudest ringtone I've ever heard in my life, but she just stares at it and doesn't know how to use it. Our other roomie just stormed over and turned it off.

4:53
They gave her something to clean her right out and she was like "Oh dear, just leave me on the bedpan. I'll let you know when it's full." So then she broke her buzzer (I suspect they disconnected it) and she yelled at me to wake up and call a nurse because she was "flowing over".

5:32
Patsy's got three guests here right now, all discussing the color of her vomit. Very loudly. I'm sat here sniggering like a 12 year old boy pretending to laugh at a magazine article. Roomie 2 looks like she's pretending to sleep, but I can see her laughing too.

5:47
It's okay. They've gone off for a "fag" now. It's just her and another Irish guy. He's actually pretty nice. Oh, she just vurped (vomited and burped at the same time). He countered by leaning to the side in his chair, lifting a bum cheek and farting loudly. Nice.

5:49
An alarm is going off. People look concerned. Am betting one of Patsy's friends fell asleep with a cigarette in the bathroom.

5:53

All the old people are very upset about the fire alarm. Bedpans are probably overflowing all over the ward right now.

9:17
Patsy just seriously told the nurse that if I'm not taking my morphine she'll have it.

In the end it was good for us, encouraging Roommate 2 and I to sneak out of the ward and to the cafeteria at meal times, though when she was discharged I was left on my own with Patsy and banned from leaving the ward. I bribed another patient to bring me up a plate of chips as my appetite returned – the chips arrived smelling lovely and steaming with warmth, salted and smothered in ketchup. I sat back in my bed and picked up a book, settling in to slowly enjoy my steaming plate of fresh, thick chips when a nurse came into the room with Patsy's lunch. I waved my arms wildly in the air at the nurse summoning her over and burst into frantic tears, begging her to give me a mere 10 minutes of peace while eating, please, *please* don't wake Patsy yet. I was so hungry. *So hungry!*

A loud vurp came from across the room with a groan. It was futile – I had woken Patsy with my frantic sobbing, and I shared a look of empathy with the nurse as I leaned over and tipped my warm plate of chips into the bin.

Damn Patsy.

Singing Gangsters and Self Esteem

I've been going to monthly chemotherapy infusions since March 2013 and am proud to say that I've made some good friends and have had some grand adventures, as well as some hard times and good laughs. There is no end to great entertainment to be found in other patients if you just approach them with a friendly smile and a sympathetic ear – and let the crazy flow where it may. It's not just entertaining but also strangely validating. The inner thoughts of crazy that you had previously kept to yourself would be espoused by other patients like these were normal conversation comments, halting you in your tracks with the realization that you are maybe neither alone nor as crazy as you had originally thought.

Anyone that has ever been on high dose prednisolone (corticosteroid) for some time knows about the steroid weight gain and Cushing's syndrome (cushingoid – sounds like some kind of star trek character) which piles on weight like nobody's business and re-distributes fat to a person's face, shoulders and stomach – giving you what is affectionately known as Moon Face Buffalo Hump. I looked like Jabba the Hut in Drag. Or maybe Egg-Man from Sonic. Either way, it's not attractive and the weight is very, very difficult to control. I knew from my experience of online forums that people struggle tremendously with self-esteem in the face of cushingoid, though I hadn't realized quite how common this was until I was in an infusion room full of other patients riddled with Rheumatoid conditions as the parade of large, perfectly round people piled in one by one to fill each chair in the room, ready for their respective infusions. We looked like a family reunion of Fisher Price Little People in there – all of us with the same perfectly round face, chubby cheeks and sunken in eyes fighting to wedge ourselves into our armchairs and sweating from the mere effort of breathing and taking off our coats. Like a pack of wounded, asthmatic hippopotami.

Then something strange yet delightful occurred, something that I had internally always wanted to do but was too afraid of coming across as some sort of vain lunatic. The woman next to me was chatting away nicely when the conversation turned, as it always does, to steroids and weight gain. "I didn't always look like this" she started, as she rustled around in her purse, triumphantly emerging with a crinkled, well-worn photo of her thin self before steroids. She thrust it toward me, "Look, look! I'm normally very thin – with great cheekbones!" To my astonishment the other steroid-round patients began to stir, producing their own pre-steroid thin pictures from wallets, purses and phones, coming together around my chair desperate to validate each other's physical condition amongst the only other people that could possibly understand.

Our diseases had changed us, our medications had altered us so irrevocably – the fatigue, the nausea, the pills to counteract the effects of all the other pills. The mania, insomnia and the crying at the toaster because it just so selfishly doesn't understand your needs. I often wish for a moment that Sarcoidosis turned a person's skin blue, so that it was at least visible when people tell you that you look well when you feel as though you are dying inside. The weight gain of Cushing's Syndrome is something that you simply cannot help, you cannot avoid. I was a wheat free vegan for God's sake! I led a healthy lifestyle and yet I looked as though I lay about all day in a flowered muumuu with the curtains drawn eating takeaway pizzas and watching daytime soap operas.

I had found… *my people*. And they were wonderful.

And then we were serenaded by a large Caribbean man, there for an infusion and covered in gold bling holding a chrome pimp cane. He stood up, crossed the room to our little crowd of steroids anonymous sufferers and belted out some top 40 song I'd vaguely heard of, then going on a long and convoluted rant about how the benefit office is screwing us all.

The crazy had commenced and all was right with the world, it was time to just sit back and enjoy.

Free tickets to Jerry Springer!

Being hooked up to a wall and an armchair you can't really escape a volatile situation to give privacy when needed. Instead you watch because really, what else is there to do? You watch like a train wreck that you cannot turn away from, like the drivers that slow when going past an accident just to witness the carnage.

I don't know *what* was going on with this day but I

started out sat in the waiting area of the Rheumatology basement – waiting my turn to see a consultant at the clinic. Many people were waiting and doctors were getting through people as fast as they could. Tempers were high and the wait was long but I rarely mind, I'm grateful to be seen and I learned to take a book (or my laptop) with me early on. (Except for at the eye hospital. Once they dilate both eyes you can't really see anything but blurry colors. I once took my laptop with me, determined to while away the hours getting some writing done, even though I couldn't see. What did it matter? I am an excellent typist – I don't need to see the keys or the screen. The next day I opened up my laptop to find that I had misplaced my hand on the keyboard one position too far left, leaving me with eight pages of complete jibberish. I must have looked like Stevie Wonder in that waiting room, staring blindly at the ceiling and waving my head around in thought, typing a wall of complete nonsense. It would have been nice had someone told me – a nudge, a creepy whispered *'your fingers are on the wrong keys'* from over my shoulder – anything.

A bit of a commotion could be heard coming from a consultant's room next to where I was sat, just a few chairs down. A man could be heard yelling at the doctor – beginning to rant and swear. The doctor was clearly trying to calm him down, being firm yet polite but this man was hell-bent on berating him for not having cured him *and* for having made him wait for so long out in the hall. The yelling got louder and other patients started looking around in alarm. Soon we were all staring at the door, wondering if a nurse or other doctor walking by would take notice and intervene – but the chatter from further down the hall was masking the severity of the sounds coming through the door.

I couldn't take it anymore, and couldn't imagine clearly needing help and nobody coming to my aid. I got up and walked round the corner to a nursing station to interrupt a male nurse on the phone. I told him as quietly as possible that it seemed as though a doctor was in trouble in the room down the hall – a patient was seeming very aggressive, perhaps someone should call security?

He thanked me and I sat back down – I could still hear the doctor being berated by this enraged man about his condition and care. I wanted to stride over and open the door, pretending to have entered the wrong room but at least getting the door open and giving the poor doctor an 'out' but kept reminding myself that as a patient that wasn't my place. But if it got worse I would do it.

The nurse came to listen at the door and did exactly that, opening the door wide and the sound of the enraged man carried through the hall, silencing everyone around as they stared. The doctor was now declining to examine or treat the man, he would have to leave and calmly return another day – this did not go over very well and about the time that security did show up the doctor had made it out of the room and the man was in there on his own, hurling things around.

My name was called just as security went in to 'remove him' from the building and I nearly opted to stay in my chair – how could I miss this!? Seriously?

Timing is rarely ever in my favor.

Luck made up for it later that day, however, with a woman sat across from me on the day-ward. This one was a real piece of work – come out of a small day surgery procedure and there for observation (why with me, I'll never know). She was a weathered woman of about fifty or so, with faded tattoos and the disposition of a drunken badger. She smiled at me and all was well, until she pulled out her phone. The woman rang a man who, after careful deduction, turned out to be her husband – though they were apparently separated at present. She complained to him, loudly, that she was all by herself in hospital after just having had surgery and why didn't he care enough to be there for her? Nobody was there for her, her own daughter wanted to come but she has the dog and the hospital wouldn't let her bring it. They just don't understand, he's a *nice* dog, pit bulls just have an unfair reputation.

I heard screaming down the other end of the line and the woman erupted, in turn screaming at her husband over the phone about his girlfriend yelling at her in the background. How dare she yell at her, she's in hospital! She didn't call the girlfriend's phone, she called her husband for support – how can he allow his girlfriend to treat his wife this way? (my eyebrows were already well up into my hairline by then). More unintelligible screaming ensued and I was tempted to send out for popcorn and a Twix.

The woman was distraught and angry, flailing around in her bed in a tantrum of fury – which resulted not in a resolution to her problems so much as her left breast somehow hanging completely out of her hospital gown without her noticing. I still don't understand how that can happen – the woman had two gowns on, one front ways and one backward – surely to ensure that all areas were appropriately covered. Right down the middle of her chest where front gown met back gown a slit had formed – perhaps an arm hole? – and her entire breast snuck out and hung there for all to see. A nurse came by and kindly pointed it out to her – I certainly wasn't going to.

An hour later, said husband actually *shows up*! He strides in dressed as a bedraggled Rastafarian and sits by her side, ever the attentive and loving husband. Except for the girlfriend that he apparently lives with. The woman loses it on him about how he can live with a woman like that and how dare he let the girlfriend yell at her over his phone. He kept trying to shut her down, glancing nervously at me (as I was sat there staring shamelessly) and telling her that they could talk about it later. She wouldn't drop it- she was like a dog with a bone. Over and around they went in a circular argument for a good hour until he shouted "ENOUGH WOMAN!" and scrounged around in her purse for change to go get himself a drink.

The husband returns to a fresh barrage of comments about the 'witch girlfriend' – her name was Evie, apparently, and how she was his *wife* and he left her for a younger woman just because the girlfriend can have sex up to five times a day and she can't. She's got things to *do*. Cue wracking sobs as she wailed to him that he made her change her name – a point which he contested vehemently.

I couldn't have asked for better roommates. This was fascinating.

More people showed up, presumably her two adult sons from another relationship. Their backstories and demeanors were equally absorbing – one complaining that the men's shelter he was living in had paper curtains for room dividers and that it was inhuman treatment. At this point I started to type away on my laptop, keen not to make eye contact should I get beaten up in a hospital – something that could really only happen to me.

The sons weren't happy about having to wait, though the woman was adamant that if she left early her lung could collapse and *didn't they care?* Doctors came and went, checked her and confirmed that she would need to wait until five to leave, the usual for post-surgical observation. The sons and husband weren't having this. One marched over to the nursing station to complain – his car was downstairs and he was double parked – why couldn't she just go now? The other had to pick up a baby. It wasn't clear whose baby it was, just that a baby needed picking up – couldn't they go now? The husband was meeting a friend (cue violent expletives from his wife about girlfriend Evie again) and she looks just fine, can't they go?

Finally, finally they were given the all-clear to help her get dressed and to go home. The wife pulled the curtain and invited the husband in to 'help her' get dressed. The other roommates and I heard a lot of sounds but not many that sounded like getting dressed, until we heard:

"Lost a lot of weight, haven't I? I'm looking good now aint I? Two and a half stone. You'd like this now, wouldn't you. Well you're not 'aving it! Not with that witch screaming at me down the phone!"

I was actually quite sad to see them leave.

Screw Triage, I was here first!

Throughout the process of being diseased I have come to enjoy the quiet sport of "people watching". Often finding myself with absolutely nothing to do and with my eyes too painfully sensitive to read I resort to observing those around me. And I'm nosy. Observing people at an airport can be a charming experience – the anticipation showing in the pacing of anxious relatives, the craning of necks and guessing where groups of passengers are from based on their dress and suitcase sizes. The teary arrivals and pure joy when finally spotted. People watching at a café can be soothing – deep conversation interspersed with light laughter, the romantic couple and, as always, the awkward first date couples. At these places you are left alone, peacefully to observe quietly, an outsider sharing in a private moment and then life quickly moving on, each flittering off in their separate ways.

Hospital people watching is not like that at all. It is not peaceful. It is not private. It is a loud, bright mess of frustration and "in your face" crazy that reaches out and lassos everyone in with drama the likes of an American high school in the waiting room of any A&E. You get the quiet sufferers in one corner, those patiently dying in their hard steel chairs of some unknown and surely communicable disease. You get the moaners – with limbs propped up and doing all they can to breathe as loudly as possible. You get the paranoid parents there to have their child's boo-boo kissed better (and *nobody* understands how serious that bruise is!) and you get the people sporting injuries so visible that the other patients recoil in horror and back away, lest a bone sticking out of your leg be catching. Of course the majority of people in the waiting room are reasonable – waiting their turn and watching the door, looking up in anticipation each time a name is called as though we are in some medical raffle, eyes turning back to the floor quietly when the name isn't ours.

And then you get the really good ones – the "MeMe's". A typical MeMe doesn't just arrive at A&E, they make an entrance. The MeMe bursts through the door as they have been racing another patient toward the entrance in a bid to get in line faster. The MeMe darts to the reception desk and clings to it in desperation, launching into a dramatic telling to the receptionist of the horror that has happened to them and requesting that they be seen as quickly as possible. The MeMe then turns around , finds a seat closest to the main doors and audibly counts the people that are "in front of them", judging (audibly) the few people they deem to be more serious than them to be the handful of people that might go in before the MeMe. The MeMe becomes increasingly vocal and offensive with each person called in before them, checking with the receptionist that something isn't wrong and wanting to know why people that arrived after them have gone in first. We've all seen a MeMe in action.

My personal favorite burst into the quiet Western Eye Hospital in London on a windy, rainy day, providing a good two hours of much needed waiting room entertainment.

An eye hospital waiting room is somewhat different from a regular hospital waiting room in that people are really only there for eye injuries, so there is less moaning and groaning than in regular hospitals. There aren't any wheelchairs or many ambulances making an appearance and, unless you are holding your eye in your hand, things tend to run along smoothly on a first come first served basis. What is even more interesting in an eye hospital waiting room, however, is the level of attention in the waiting room. We can barely see, and then dilating drops are put into our eyes so then we *really* can't see anything. Just blurs and colors and people if they are far enough away. We cannot read books, play on our phones, read the newspaper or even read the dull leaflets dispersed throughout the room. So we sit there and watch each other rather shamelessly – all with the understanding that there is really nothing else to do.

So when the doors to the A&E burst open with a bang

and in flew a tall woman in an oversized full fur coat purposefully striding to the reception, twenty-three heads all turned and spirits brightened – finally we would have something worth watching. Oh, and how we did.

The woman, middle aged and very loud, re-enacted her ordeal in a sharp, nasal American accent to the poor receptionist, who had only asked for her name and date of birth. We listened, captivated, as she told us of treachery at a small London theater. She had been sitting in the audience, having paid good money (good money I tell you!) for her seat at a certain play by a Director she had much respect for, when a theater fan blew a great cloud of debris off the stage and *into the audience*. She had felt something fly directly into her eye and experienced excruciating pain, screaming in her seat until they finally stopped the play to care for her appropriately. She couldn't believe the nerve of the ushers asking her to go out into the hall – she couldn't walk around, she had an eye injury!

The play was stopped and a flashlight was shone into her eye but nothing was found – of course nothing was found, she needed urgent medical treatment as it had clearly *gone into her eye* and insisted that they call her an ambulance, at their cost and to send her to a private hospital, also at the theater's cost. The theater called an ambulance and was turned down as it was "not an emergency requiring an ambulance" with the advice to go to an eye hospital on her own. On her own! Didn't anyone *care*? She was nearly blind! And the theater! They should be ashamed of themselves! (at this point the receptionist was asking her repeatedly to please sit down, save it for the doctor) The woman, oblivious to the captivated audience behind her (this was amazing! One woman was called and she shushed the doctor, waving him off in favor of finishing the dramatic re-enactment of the irate American woman) continued her tale of woe, appealing to the receptionist's sympathies that she had to come here on her own and at her own expense even, surely the receptionist could *at least* ensure that she is seen quickly as she has already endured so much, so much!

The elaborately fur clad woman finally turned to find a chair as we all quickly averted our eyes and again pretended to play with the phones we couldn't see, half hoping that she wouldn't sit beside us but then again half hoping that she would. The woman's hair was short and wild, her makeup looked as though it had been applied with some sort of makeup shotgun from 1987. She sat down into an empty steel chair with a huff and a comment about the waiting room being too crowded and then immediately turned to the near blind gentleman beside her to ask him, loudly, how one would go about finding a personal injury lawyer at the hospital as that theater deserves to be sued and shut down.

Doctors came and went through their swinging double doors of mystery – where patients entered but never came out. Still our names weren't called. The waiting room emptied and filled with a constant trickle of near-blind patients bumping into things and apologizing to the gurgling water cooler and empty chairs. Every single time a name was called that wasn't hers the MeMe huffed and puffed and scoffed and tskd and got up to check that the receptionist hadn't forgotten to put her chart into the pile. She checked how many people were before her and harassed the triage nurse for not having competently grasped her level of pain that she was enduring in the waiting room, compared to all of these other people "who look just fine!" She threatened to go to another eye hospital. She advised us all to sue. And when an elderly woman who arrived after her was called in before her this woman pitched a fit, jumping out of her chair and cutting off the elderly near blind woman in the aisle. She made it to the doctor and demanded that she be seen right this instant as she had been waiting the longest of anyone in this room (aside from about eight of us who had been there longer than she but were just much less vocal about it) The doctor silenced her with a look of steel and the MeMe meekly returned to her seat to rant instead to her captive audience of other waiting patients.

The doors swung open and a name was called, I'd gotten so used to the disappointment that I had more or less stopped listening – nearly missing my own name. It was my turn, finally. As I stood the American woman glared at me from her chair, as it was clearly my fault that I was called in before her. As I passed I heard her mutter to the people next to her that I looked fine, why should I go in before her?

So I turned to her, removed my oversized sunglasses and opened my blood red eyes wide, looking like something out of a zombie movie to glare at her – the full force of the zombie death stare unleashed upon this poor woman and the others around her without warning. She recoiled in horror as I smiled, turned and limped up the aisle moaning "braaaaains…. braaaaaains….." which she didn't think was particularly funny – though the waiting ophthalmologist was busting a gut laughing.

Sometimes you've just got to have some fun with it.

Chapter Four: Welcome to the Funny Farm

I've always wondered why hospital admissions don't come with a Welcome Pack, or at least an instruction manual of some sort. Being admitted, especially from the emergency department, is an odd experience that we, as patients, know very little about and in which we can control absolutely nothing. It starts with a wristband being slapped on and everything suddenly moving very fast, as though you are instantly no more than a spectator of your own experience. Nurses start bustling about gathering your things and, if you are Canadian like me, the shoes I took off before putting my feet up on the bed (getting it dirty would be rude!) are thrust into a plastic HAZMAT bag along with your purse, coat and laptop (oh, you don't bring a laptop with you to A&E in case something funny happens? Just me?) and out of nowhere a man with a wheelchair is at the door tapping his foot impatiently and expecting you to get in.

Where are we going? What's going on? Who is *this* guy? Wait... is all you can squeak out amongst the bustle of doctors coming in and out to poke you and write things in charts while a nurse holding a blue bag of your worldly possessions forcefully helps you into said wheelchair. You are then told that you are being admitted (so I'm not going home for dinner then?), assured that a cheese sandwich will be found somewhere and wheeled away down the hall clutching that god-awful blue bag.

My legs aren't broken. I've not passed out nor am I dizzy, but they never let me walk to the ward. It's a rule, you have to go up by wheelchair or bed. Even when I was there for eye problems. You could break your arm and they would still stick you into that wheelchair. So you sit back and let your cheeks flush with embarrassment as you are wheeled along the "transfer of shame", clutching that ridiculous blue bag. First it is out of your little room in A&E as all of the other patients stare at you with a mix of pity and envy – you are at least going *somewhere*. They look at your legs, which are clearly not broken, and wonder why you are being wheeled about. No matter, they are gone in seconds as you whizz down the hall. Into the main corridor of the hospital crowded with patients, staff and the worst – visitors. The patients and the staff understand. They've seen the forced wheelchair transfer of shame themselves. They know it's not your fault. The visitors don't, though. They glance down to your unbroken legs and then back up to your perfectly healthy looking self, forcing this exhausted looking gentleman to push you around the hospital like a spoiled hypochondriac. I feel my cheeks flush and call back to the porter that I don't mind walking, but he ignores me and continues on his speed trial of hallway maneuvers.

We come to a door and I am compelled to "help" by trying to hold the door open for him, while in the wheelchair, and nearly launch myself out onto the floor, whacking the side of my head with the door and spilling the contents of my bag – barely catching the laptop but the bra I had to take off during an earlier chest x-ray and couldn't be bothered to put back on goes skittering across the floor. I sink back into the chair with eyes wide and face bright red as the porter collects my bra from down the hall, brings it back to me and firmly assures me that my help is not needed. I am also suddenly again aware that I am not wearing a bra and wondering if *that* is what people were staring at in the hall.

Fine. Open your own damn doors then. Ohhhhh. They're automatic.

Damn.

We then get to the ward and I tell the porter again that I don't mind walking from here, I would quite like to stretch my legs anyway. He's not having it, especially after that whole flying bra incident, so I am wheeled right to a bedside and forced to climb directly from the wheelchair to the abnormally high bed without the use of a solid floor. He's not taking any chances with me and before my bum is firmly on that bed he's out of there, off to humiliate another perfectly mobile, helpful person I'm sure.

Nurses then come in with small talk and assurances, I'm told to relax and we again go over what medications I am on, a cheese sandwich is again mentioned and I am continuously told to relax – there is nothing more I can do than to wait quietly, the doctors will be doing their rounds shortly. No you can't go home, no you cannot order in Dominoes Pizza. Still no when I offered to order some for the nursing station too.

The nurses on the ward are outstandingly busy and the quick squeak of their sneakers over the floor never stops, I don't want to take up their time and assure them that I am alright, I will wait here. I promise I won't get up and move about, nor will I order in a Chinese. I won't unplug the IV thing to plug in my laptop and I won't go downstairs in search of that elusive cheese sandwich. And so I sit, quietly and alone, listening to the beeps and the sounds of the ward and I wait. I don't even know what I'm waiting for, but I wait, and I am happy and grateful to do so.

I once had a profound moment at Hammersmith Hospital in London – when I had been admitted on Thanksgiving with Bell's Palsy and a crazy flare (my first), in which I quietly sobbed in my dark little room after the flurry of being admitted. Hearing me crying a nurse quietly came into my room, sat on the corner of my bed and took my hand. She didn't say anything - she didn't have to. She couldn't promise everything would be okay, none of us knew what was happening to me. But she held my hand and told me that they would take care of me.

And in that moment I didn't feel so alone, I would be okay.

Being an in-patient in hospital is a frightening experience full of unknown and a complete loss of control. You are at the full mercy of those that care for you and the only real choices you get to make are menu items and whether or not you will go to the bathroom now or try to see how long you can hold it, just for something to do. We are at the full mercy of student doctors, transport breakdowns and a schedule that is not for the faint of heart (or those suffering from drug induced paranoia – *that* was fun as well). You've really just got to roll with it, go with the flow and enjoy the ride.

But an instruction manual would have been nice.

The Bed Pan Incident

I was in my hospital ward, surrounded by elderly women of both the gentle and senile variety, having just come back from a bronchoscopy – a simple procedure in which a bunch of people wearing masks and gloves partly sedate you and shove a tube down your throat and into your lungs to take a biopsy. The day-surgeon rushed over to me in the recovery area of the procedure ward, anxious with his good news that it wasn't cancer, it was non-caseating granulomas (whatever *that* was) – and that this was looking more and more like Sarcoidosis. (I still didn't know what that was at the time, but it sounded better than cancer so I was happy).

Having mulled it over for a day, my team of specialists at the hospital felt that a further biopsy was still needed, my Bell's Palsy hadn't yet subsided and a biopsy of a gland in my face would be the second confirmation they needed to move forward with treatment. I only found this out when a nurse came with a wheelchair, ready with transport to take me to another hospital for the procedure. Cue another bout of frantic panicking, my husband being called and him dashing off to meet me at the next hospital, bringing with him my boss and best friends. It was an odd group, but I appreciated having them there.

I remember being wheeled away in my hospital bed hyperventilating from stress and sure that this was about to be the end of me. Surgeons surrounded my bed outside of the operating room, looking down on me in a circle of concerned faces obscured in the harsh lights above. They seemed very concerned about the potential for permanent damage to the nerves in my face though I assured them, through my newly acquired pirate-themed Bell's Palsy accent, that whatever they did couldn't be much worse than the position I was already in. We all had a bit of a chuckle (mine was a rather high pitched nervous squeak) and I felt myself drift away to sleep.

And then I had to pee.

I remember this intense need to relieve myself as I struggled to open my eyes (well, eye. Only one was working at the time) and found myself in the recovery room, hooked up to beeping monitors and bags of liquid. I felt for all of my limbs, everything seemed intact. I'd survived. This was good. But I really, really had to pee. I tried calling for a nurse, but my throat was sore and raspy. I really, *really* needed to pee. Thankfully, a nurse heard my incessant croaking and rushed over to check on me, assuring me that everything had gone well (though my arms and hands seemed to be covered in many more IV's and holes than I remember going in with) and I asked her where I might find the bathroom. She looked at me, puzzled, and gently explained that I wasn't to get out of bed. Although I agreed, given how unsteady I was feeling just lying there, I assured her that we were approaching a crisis here and told her that I could feel my kidneys floating around. She gave me a bedpan.

I was appalled, and confided to her in an unintentionally loud whisper that I didn't have a clue how to use a bedpan, it would really just be easier for everybody if she unhooked me and pointed me toward the loo.

She left me hooked up, with the bedpan. I croaked for her to come back, I don't know how to use this thing! Rolling her eyes (understandably), she returned to deftly and expertly slip the cold bedpan under my bottom, pulled the curtain around me for privacy and then left me to it.

And I didn't have a clue what to do about it.

Tears sprung to my eyes as I lay there in the most awkward position ever, lying flat on my back with my hips and bum up in the air, sure I was going to just wet myself. Already in a hospital gown with nothing between myself and the cold, hard bedpan I figured all I would have to do is just let it go and it would surely happen.

It didn't.

You just can't pee like that, it's not natural. Even just lying there, resigning myself to just go, nothing happened. I must have been doing something wrong. Maybe you had to sit on it. Clearly that's what I had to do. Just sit on it. I tried, but my arms and legs weren't quite doing what I was telling them to do. In trying to sit up my arm flung out and smashed into the bed rail, causing a ruckus as I called out "I'm fine!" over the curtain before the nurse could burst in and see what I was doing. After a few minutes of gripping the bed rails to pull myself into a sitting position I was finally there, sitting on this cold hard thing with my legs straight out in front of me. Still nothing. We're simply not designed to pee while sitting up with your legs straight out in front of you. It just doesn't work like that.

Maybe I had to kneel over it or something. Okay, I could do that. I was thinking that it would have been much easier to just walk to the bathroom at this point, but the nurse wouldn't unhook me and I'm always terrified to do anything that might dislodge a needle (that arm was dead to me). By that time I was on my hospital bed, in a gown and wobbling around on my hands and knees trying to maneuver myself over this stupid bedpan, near to bursting with urine and desperation. Maybe I should just pee the bed. That would show her.

This clearly wasn't working. I had to stand up over this thing. It was the only way, and I was beyond desperate. I gripped the rail with my one good hand and pushed myself up onto my feet, slowly rising to a wobbly standing position and closed my eyes in relief as I experienced the sweet relief of final success. The rushing noise of the stream hitting the bedpan caused the nurses at their station to turn until they saw me, head sticking out above the curtain standing on my bed to pee all over the bed pan as I glared and shouted: "I told you I didn't know how to use this thing!"

Paying back the NHS in Guinea Pig Tax

Something that I have come to notice with having a rare condition is the amount of interest it seems to generate, especially in a teaching hospital. Not only are doctors seemingly interested as it must be nice to see something new once in a while, but so are nurses, specialists and even pharmacists. The catering staff were much more difficult to impress - and did not feel that my rare condition warranted an extra trifle pudding with dinner.

It would always start with an A&E doctor slowly realizing what he or she was seeing and putting in a call to Rheumatology. My file would be fetched and, while waiting, student or junior doctors would start arriving to "just have a look". They would ask me the same questions, do the same exams and marvel at my medical history. Ask about medications, family history and just how it is my eyes turned *that* grotesque shade of red. A Rheumatologist would arrive with another student in tow, no doubt quickly pulled off their ward duties so as not to miss this opportunity. Once they find out that I'm pretty nice and easy going it then starts to go a bit overboard – me being admitted is like a field day for medical students around London as I've come to find.

Once the crisis is over and dealt with I am often approached by a senior doctor or someone on my medical team asking me if I would mind if some of their students could come in to see me, examine me, ask me questions or go over my medical history. My answer has always been the same, it's not like I have anything better to do in here, why not? Sometimes they would wink and ask me not to tell the students what I have – better for them to come up with it themselves, which they did desperately and frantically – the first to come up with it running out of the room in unabashed glee to find their senior doctor with the diagnosis, the others hot on their heels.

My personal favorite was a young rheumatologist in A&E who, after countless other doctors had come in to see me and left with no clear diagnosis, took a quick look at me in the darkened A&E room, consulted his iPhone App and came up with Sarcoidosis, something he had heard about in med school at one point. It turns out he was right, though we didn't know that yet. His bedside manner needed work but I loved him – a fresh doctor that was compassionate and attentive. You just couldn't help but have a lot of faith in this guy. Once I was admitted and brought onto a ward I remember sitting up in bed on painkillers so strong I was seeing unicorns prancing along the outer hall, with the right side of my face paralyzed and my eyes a burning red. He meekly sat on the foot of my bed, arms loaded with paperwork, and told me that he realized that this probably wasn't the best timing, but he really thinks this is a fascinating presentation and he would love to use my case as a medical study – could I please sign these permission forms for the British Medical Journal? And this one, and this one… and this one….

Why not? It's not like I had anything else to do.

It is funny how things come full circle, as two and a half years later I saw that doctor again, and still see him now as one of my primary care providers. He is now working exclusively under a Sarcoidosis specialist in London. I'm not sure if I should take that as a compliment or not, but it is a bit strange to have a degree of disease so rare and interesting that it changes the career path of your A&E doctor.

I once had gone to my GP for an open surgery appointment at which she got all excited and called in her medical student, a young Chinese guy with eagerness written all over his face. She told him, in front of me, that in all his years as a doctor he would be lucky to ever see a case like this and he looked me up and down like I was a piece of meat at a butchers. She asked him what he thought my diagnosis was, just by looking at me (not quite possible but hey, let her have some fun with the poor kid). I stood up and he walked around me once, slowly, measuring me up and down and then, pointing right at me loudly declared "Moon Face, Buffalo Hump! You must be on high dose steroids as you are so very large, your face is so perfectly round and you have a hunchback upon your shoulders."

Oh. Um, thanks.

I just can't win

Doctors seem to be a big fan of "pain scales", in which you are asked to rate your pain from 0 to 10, 0 being non-existent (so why would you be here?) and 10 being the worst pain you have ever felt in your life (wouldn't you likely be dead?). I personally think that they make an adjustment of 3 to account for hypochondria and general melodrama, so that if you say 10 it's really a 7 and if you say 2 it's really a -1 so they smack you upside the head for wasting their time and someone goes off to call you a minicab.

I like to think that I have a high tolerance for pain (who doesn't like to think that?) but I have learned, through the course of being diseased, that the more pain you endure the more you learn to handle, twisted and sadistic as that sounds. Actually it sounds like the ad for a brothel in Amsterdam, but we don't need to go there. Over the last two and a half years I have had some serious doozies, the flares causing searing pain to the point of paralysis and slipping in and out of consciousness.

I remember one point, where things were particularly awful. I was in so much pain in my bones that even the slightest touch felt like being hit with a sledgehammer. I would scream out at the brush of a hand against my knee or even the thought of putting shoes on my feet. I could stand, but I couldn't handle being touched. It felt as though my bones were in a vice grip being crushed until the point that they wouldn't be able to take any more and would burst into dust. I've been brought in to hospital a couple of times like this, and it is a terrible thing to try to explain but also a terrible thing to endure the poking and prodding of tests. Steroid infusions usually fix me right up but they always have to be sure it isn't something else, first. So in I go, usually for a long stay.

In my two and a half years with this thing this was the worst I had ever felt. The pain was too much to bear and, even lying still, the stabbing, crushing pain in my bones caught my breath in my throat. I would pour with sweat, soaking my hair and clothes – then suddenly freeze in my wet bed, clutching a heating pad to my chest and willing it to warm up my very heart, shivering with fever. The temperature controls of my body had gone haywire with the flare. My eyes were bloody red and I couldn't bear to open them in the light. The right side of my face had fallen again with a searing pain and the hardening of the right side of my neck. It was so dark and there was nothing to focus on but the pain and the fear and the cold. There was a moment, as I lay there in agony and desperation, that I felt I could just… go. Just let go and it would be over, just let my heart stop beating and my lungs stop lifting. Let go and be at peace, just let it go. Like it was suddenly a choice, a choice that I could just make and be done with it.

I wasn't ready. I will be, one day, but not now. It would be better, and Paul would be here soon. I wasn't alone – I just needed some help. And some very powerful drugs.

I remember one of these times in particular, and being asked to rate my pain on the pain scale. Now, my GP has warned me before about my demeanor and being taken seriously in an A&E, as she understands the severity of things and that I usually need to be seen quite quickly. She explained that the overweight, non-complaining, patient and cheery woman sat in the waiting room is going to be bumped to the bottom of the list whereas if I were to let it out properly things may go a bit more in my favor, but I just can't do it. I can't be that waiting room screamer – even when I was having a stroke. So I mask my pain with bad jokes and apologies for taking up their time, not always the best A&E strategy but hey, at least I'm interesting.

Remembering the pain scale and rule of three I was feeling probably a nine but I told them an eight, just in case. I didn't want to appear too dramatic. For the first time the doctor and nurses stopped what they were doing, looked at me in surprise and said "Really? Are you sure? Because we can feel the heat coming off your shins and face." to which I responded with something lame about not wanting to appear melodramatic and I'm so sorry about taking up so much of everyone's time. The pain then got much worse and I started rambling as a cannula was put into my arm and some morphine pumped in. A doctor was stood by my side asking me standard intake questions about medications and what I was feeling and then he asked me my name – I told him, Candace (in my Canadian accent with a bit of a Bell's Palsy drawl). He looked puzzled and asked me to repeat my name again. Candace. Cayn-dayce. Candace.

He looked downright alarmed as he checked out my records – he asked the nurses my name – Candeese, they said in their British accents. Her name is Candeese, not Cayn-dayce.

It was determined that, as I was apparently saying my own name incorrectly, I was too far gone and I was shot up with something that put me to sleep.

I woke up in a ward hours later sweating and panting in the pain of the flare. A nurse darted back over and asked me my name. Cayn-dayce. In went the shot before I could realize what the issue was and I was out.

I woke the next day to the same nurse standing by my bedside, needle in hand. Before she could ask me my name I burst out that I was Canadian, the problem wasn't my name, it was my accent! Well, that and my face wasn't quite working the way it normally does. She looked skeptical. The pain in my legs and face started to rear up as I was about to explain the whole Cayn-dayce / Candeese accent thing when she again asked me my name. I thought about it for a split second… oh, what the hell.

Cayn-dayce.

Bliss.

Does an Echocardiogram count as being felt up if it was by a really hot doctor?

At one point I was very new to all this. I had no idea what any of these tests were, I thought my GP referring me to a Rheumatologist meant that I had bone cancer and that an echocardiogram was some sort of hearing test. I was even more shocked to find out what an "internal ultrasound" was, but that is an experience for another day. Shudder.

I've since gone to support groups for Sarcoidosis and now appear so knowledgeable about this disease, treatments, specialists and tests that other patients have assumed that I was surely a doctor myself. I'll admit that I didn't quite correct them until after they had bought me dinner and a drink, but I feel that it is nearly impossible to go through something like this without picking up as much information along the way as you can. So I pride myself now on being a source of knowledge and support to others with my condition or similar conditions, and take part in an online forum as well as a London support group (which is entertaining as all hell, but probably not for the right reasons) – and am proud that others have found me online and have struck up contact in person (like stalkers?) for support and guidance.

Because when I started with this thing I knew *nothing*. And I mean nothing. I was a hapless, cheerful (until the internal ultrasound) idiot just going along for the ride and hoping for the best. I would be scheduled a test and have no idea what it was for, how it would happen or how long it would take. My only concerns were about whether or not it was going to hurt or whether I should wear my lululemon yoga pants for the test and then change at work or just try to get away with wearing yoga pants at work all day afterward.

So my husband started coming to these things with me because really, someone has to pay attention.

Neither of us really knew what an echocardiogram was, except that we had googled it a bit and it turned out to be some kind of ultrasound of the heart. Probably really quick, no big deal. Definitely wear the yoga pants and maybe don't eat anything an hour beforehand, just in case. We arrived at the Echocardiogram area and were called in almost immediately – I was given a gown to change into by the female technician and she left the room, promising to be back in a moment to get things started. My husband helped me change into the gown, no big deal (I kept my yoga pants on) and I perched on the bed/table thing in wait while my husband sat on the chair beside the table sipping his coffee and cracking jokes about my flimsy hospital gown.

The female tech came back with a few forms for me to sign and that was, apparently, the last we were going to see of her as she walked out and Adonis walked in.

He was tall. Tanned. Thick, curly blonde hair that fell past his ears. Muscular and ruggedly handsome with the kind of chiseled jaw you only see in men's underwear ads. He opened his mouth and wow! Australian!

Swoon! He looked like he belonged on a surfboard and was rocking those scrubs like nobody's business. I blushed, glancing to my husband who was trembling with silent giggles.

The tech sat down in his swivel chair beside me, explained that we were going to check out my heart and look for any holes (wait, what?) and then they were going to inject some dye and do it again (wait, what?). The whole thing should only take about 45 minutes (what?) and could I please take off my gown and roll toward him (wait, WHAT?). I glanced to my husband again who was absolutely dying in his chair with silent giggles at my predicament.

Here's the thing about me – I laugh when I am uncomfortable. And I am uncomfortable a lot. It comes out as completely inappropriate laughter and I cannot stop. I start giggling and then I'm done, there is no coming back from the giggles when they start. It's not a charming, disarming social quality. It just makes everything that much more uncomfortable.

So the technician turned off the lights and I did what I was told, disrobed and sucked in my stomach as far as it would go. The only light was from the ultrasound monitor, giving off an eerie blue mood lighting. All we needed was some 1970's guitar and a video camera and we could probably make some good money off of this. We then proceeded to what has been the strangest exam I have ever undergone with warmed up gel and my chest being manhandled by an outrageously gorgeous Australian while my husband looked on, laughing hysterically at my increasing discomfort. I started laughing and the tech got angry – too much stuff was bouncing around and "this is hahdly a veray funny situaation madam" was scolded more than once. Another tech came in to shoot me up with dye and then the fun really started, with one person lifting and the other person scanning, my husband howling with laughter and tears pouring down his cheeks – me dying of mortification on the table but relieved that due to the dark the technicians couldn't see my bright red cheeks.

By the end of it I felt as though I should have left some sort of a tip.

Or my phone number.

If you want something done correctly...

There are few things in life as complicated, frustrating, infuriating or soul-destroying than hospital transport. Intra-hospital transport (bringing patients between multiple hospitals) is even worse, and takes only slightly less multiple department coordination than building, launching and landing a Mars Rover. Patients don't make things much easier either – with the amount of deafness, awkward positioning and general senility of transport patients I assume it is quite similar to trying to not only herd cats but then teach them algebra once you've got them. Ambulance transfers? Not a problem. But those external transport companies are an adventure not for the faint of heart.

My saga of hospital transport woe and adventure

occurred at my diagnosis visit – the very long 13 day hospital stay of darkened rooms, mental roommates and countless tests. My case was not an easy one and required specialists – but they weren't here. These specialists were dispersed throughout London at various hospitals and only the best would do for this type of thing. They made it sound as though procedures at their own hospital were performed by recovering circus monkeys but whatever, I'm sure they had their reasons and, as always, I think the NHS is an amazing system and I am eternally grateful to it. I've just had some unexpected fun along the way.

Hospital transport seems to work on the principle of spontaneity and surprise. If a patient isn't expecting it they can't moan if it doesn't show up, nor can they spend an entire day moaning about it probably not showing up and checking at the nurse's station constantly to see if it has arrived. So I get it. I wouldn't tell people beforehand either. One minute you are sitting in your hospital bed playing the "I wonder how long I can hold my pee" game and the next a guy is at the door with a wheelchair telling you to grab your coat. It's fun! A nurse then follows in with your giant binder of notes in a sealed plastic bag (for me to carry but not peek!) and tells me that I'm going over to St. Mary's Hospital for a hearing test.

"A hearing what?"

"A hearing test. HEARING TEST"

"I'm not deaf, why are you shouting at me?"

"You need a hearing test. At St. Mary's. We don't do them here."

"What?"

"A HEARING TEST"

"Yes, I heard you. Where are we going?"

"Just get in the chair."

So I am wheeled down, in my yoga pants and not having brushed my teeth (I had been saving that to give myself something to do in the afternoon) I was brought to a room on the ground floor of the hospital to sit amongst the others waiting for transport. Aside from the guy without any legs I was easily the youngest one in there by a good 30 years and the only one still wearing a hospital gown as a shirt. Bah, it was a warm summer day, what did I care? I was put into the back of a minivan and elderly patients were piled in like we were some sort of clown car. They didn't know where they were going either but I figured that might be par for the course for a couple of them anyway.

All I know is that I am meant to be going to another hospital for another test or procedure so I am really just along for the ride. We started dropping people off… at their homes. Throughout London. Just driving around in a black van in a hospital gown dropping off old people at homes they didn't always recognize. We got to the last elderly lady and she not only needed help getting to the door but to get in and upstairs as well – to which the driver kindly obliged. For a while.

I'm normally a pretty patient and easy going person, but after a few minutes of waiting I noticed that my arm was feeling a bit… wet. I looked at my bandaged club of a hand, nothing looked out of the ordinary. I should probably check it out, though. So I started to slowly unravel the white gauze around my hand and forearm, being careful to ball it back up so I could quickly re-wrap it before the driver noticed. Alarmingly near the bottom layers there was a bit of dark red – was I *bleeding*!? In the back of a black van in the midst of some kind of British senior's village? How far were we from the hospital?! I kept going, unraveling it completely to assess the damage. The tube taped to my arm from the cannula line was filled to the tip with dark red blood – *my* dark red blood. Was it *supposed* to do that? I didn't think so, and started to panic. Something had jarred and a thin line of blood was trickling out from under the tape surrounding the needle. I was very sure that wasn't meant to happen, nor was it a good thing.

Where the hell was that driver???

Okay, this was bad. Tube filled with blood and something was clearly wrong with the needle. This was not good. No sign of driver – he had gone in with the elderly woman and closed the door. They were probably having tea, oblivious to the bleeding woman still in the back of his van. I stared at the door, willing the driver to come out. I debated calling the hospital on my mobile to somehow get the driver's phone number, but realized that probably wouldn't even be possible. Where *was* he? I was about to have a medical emergency over here!

I would have to go and get him.

Now, I have gotten some strange looks before in my life. I've deserved most of them, too. But there is little stranger than a person, in the middle of a council estate, lurching out of a black, unmarked van in a flimsy hospital gown with a bandaged up club-arm and squinting in the sunlight like an elated escapee. Hospital gown flapping behind me in the breeze I limped to the door, club arm held high in the air (higher than my heart!) and banged on the woman's door, waiting impatiently on the step – suddenly very aware of doors and windows being opened suspiciously all along the street. A small crowd had started to gather near the van, staring up at me in shocked silence. The door finally opened and the hassled looking driver's mouth fell open as I snapped "I don't know what you're doing in there, but I'm bleeding, a lot. It's starting to look like a crime scene in your van. Can we go!?"

My next adventure with hospital transport, same stay and same ward – started out just as usual with a surprise guy with a wheelchair at the door and a nurse saying that I was due for a heart monitor to be fitted, again at St. Mary's. Again, nothing better to do as I was more or less a hospital captive already by that point so off I went, holding the blue bag of notes and at least thinking to swap my hospital gown for a clean t-shirt this time. I still had on my wristbands and my cannula was wrapped up into another arm-club (I was assured that it wouldn't bleed through this time) and off I went into the black, unmarked car with a stressed out driver and an elderly woman who was also going for heart monitoring at St. Mary's.

We arrived and followed the driver up to the designated area for "in patients of other hospitals" which was only slightly nicer than the general outpatients area in that they gave us cups of water, had a TV tuned to *Cash in the Attic* and wouldn't let us leave by ourselves. The driver registered both myself and the elderly woman at the desk and we sat back to wait and learn all about how the odd cheap looking paintings in our attics (doesn't everybody find old paintings in their attic?) are most likely the work of Van Gough and we should really contact the BBC to have them checked. Personally, in all my global flat renting adventures the coolest things I have found left in flats have been an assortment of mismatched shoes and a Mongolian sword hidden in my bed, but those are stories for another day.

We waited. Other people came and went. We continued to wait. The elderly woman was called up and didn't come back. I continued to wait. I checked at the desk, are you sure my name is on there? Are you sure they are expecting me? Oh yes, he says. They've got my file. I just need to wait.

So I wait. I tire quickly of *Cash in the Attic* and resort to people watching, making up wild backstories the like to suit the assortment of "in-patients from other hospitals" in their gowns and with their shortages of limbs. I soon tired of that too and, having nearly resolved to sit back and have a nap in my chair like a narcoleptic senior my phone rang – it was my husband, Paul.

"Where are you?!? Are you okay?!?"

"What? Yes, I'm fine. Why wouldn't I be? I'm just sat here dying of old age waiting for a heart test. Are *you* okay?"

"The nurses on your ward called me – they can't find you! Where are you?!"

"What? I'm where they sent me!"

Apparently not. Transport brought me to the wrong hospital completely – I was meant to be at Charing Cross, not here. The staff at my hospital were losing their brains as the transport company had no record of bringing me anywhere after having picked me up, Charing Cross had no record of me arriving and for all they knew I had been kidnapped and my organs were about to be harvested and sold. As a last ditch resort they, not actually having *my* number, called my emergency contact (husband) to tell him that A: they had lost me and B: could he help them to find me?

So he called, I answered and he gave me the number for the ward at Hammersmith – who were *very* relieved to hear from me and even more pleased that I found the whole situation rather funny. Transport was booked to take me from St. Mary's back to my bed at Hammersmith as the heart monitoring department of Charing Cross had now closed for the night anyway.

And the driver wouldn't even stop to get a takeaway on the way back. Different driver, same company. That guy was not letting me out of his sight and took me, by the arm, from his car right into the hospital. He held my arm even in the elevator and literally handed me to a ward nurse who nearly burst into tears upon seeing me back at the desk.

Shame he'd forgotten to bring back my notes.

Transport's Last Stand

I was now nine days in to the hospital stay from hell. I'd had an assortment of crazies coming and going – like the midnight wellies creeper from Room 3 – I had been traumatized and lost by hospital transport on two separate occasions and had developed a twisted love affair for hospital macaroni and cheese that was suspiciously lacking in macaroni. There wasn't much more that could go wrong, surely.

The Rheumatology team had been excited the day before with the prospect of shoving a tube down my lungs to see what they might find. Again, the procedure couldn't be done here (what *could* be done here?) and I was again off to St. Mary's for a bronchoscopy. I would be heading over there later today, sometime in the early afternoon for a quick procedure and then would be brought back straight away – nothing to worry about.

Except that transport didn't come.

They didn't come at all. The early afternoon came and went. The late afternoon arrived and still no transport. The nurse in charge, a rather jumpy man, came by a few times to rant about transport and how this wasn't *his* fault and that he has called them again and they are on their way. They didn't come that day – after a full day of waiting and yet another seemingly unnecessary day in captivity for me. Not to worry I was told, transport would pick me up first thing in the morning and I would be off and back in no time.

Again, transport didn't come. The jumpy nurse in charge was irate. Someone at the bronchoscopy side of St. Mary's was equally annoyed and the procedure was re-scheduled again, for the next day. Yet another wasted day of captivity, this was getting to be too much. The next morning came and went, still no transport. It wasn't really funny anymore – I had two young children that missed their mother and a job that seriously needed me back. Transport delays had just caused me an extra two completely unnecessary days of hospital captivity and I was starting to get upset. I might even complain and hey, I'm Canadian! We don't normally *do* that.

It was mid-afternoon when the nurse in charge told me, again, that transport wasn't coming and the procedure would have to be again re-scheduled. No way. I confirmed with him that the hospital was ready for me, right? I just had to get there and come back, right? Yes, he said, but there was no way to do it.

I could take a taxi.

No, that wasn't okay – I had to have someone with me and they couldn't let me go off alone, nor could they send nurses around London in taxis with patients.

Fine. My husband will drive me.

He paused in thought and I saw my opening. It's fine, I don't mind at all. My husband can come to the ward, pick up me and my notes, sign any waivers they want and drive me directly to St. Mary's. Then he could pick me up afterward and bring me right back here. We cut transport out of the process completely, get the procedure done and make it back to Hammersmith in time for dinner – not a big deal at all. You guys let me go out with him to the park across the street – it's just like that, no big deal. Like a day pass.

I could see the wheels turning in his head. He would go to make some calls and I quickly called Paul to get over here and explained the plan. He would pick me up from the ward, drive me to another hospital for some kind of surgery and then drive me back – no big deal. He wasn't all that comfortable with the idea but he wanted a diagnosis as badly as I did so he dropped the kids off at a friend's place and rushed over.

The deal struck with the hospital was that a nurse from my ward had to take me to my car and hand my notes to my husband, who would sign for them *and* me. He would drive me there, call this number when we arrived and a nurse would again collect me from the car and bring me to the ward. Same thing on the way back, no stopping for dinner or drinks in between.

We grabbed a nurse and bolted for the door before anyone could change their mind.

All in all we got to St. Mary's just fine, on time and the procedure went well, though I came out of it very drowsy and keen to get back to my hospital bed at Hammersmith. A nurse told me that I would be able to go soon, could I text my husband to go to the loading area?

Twenty minutes later and I was still in the recovery room. Something had to be checked and we weren't yet ready to go. I texted my husband about the delay. Another twenty minutes and we still weren't ready, the doctor hasn't yet written in my notes. (maybe he could just email something over later?). Texted husband and got a rather curt response back. Now, it wasn't *my* fault that this was taking so long. I was doing what I could to hurry it up but really, what could I actually do? He was miffed that I told him to go to the loading area and wait – a parking warden was very annoyed with him and would be back shortly – could we please get a move on? The nurse assured me that we would be going soon, not to worry. It had been an hour, he had been sitting at the loading area for an hour!

I was starting to panic – I felt terrible making him wait

like this, I shouldn't have texted him that we were ready. Why couldn't this go any faster? I felt fine, the nurse was there – surely we could just grab the notes and go? Did we really need the notes anyway? Maybe the notes could be sent over later? The nurse assured me that we were nearly ready to go probably another five minutes or so. I texted my husband – five minutes.

Fifteen minutes later I was still sat there, sorely regretting having texted my husband that we would be coming out soon and starting to understand why the hospital didn't like to tell me about transport until they were actually there. He was getting annoyed. Not at me, at the general situation and parking wardens in London can be very frightening people. We just needed to *go*. It had gone on much later than anticipated – it was already nearly seven o'clock and he had been sitting at the loading area since about five thirty. This was getting ridiculous. Could we *please* go? Please?

Wha-ha! The notes were ready, the nurse had her coat on and we were good to go – texted husband that we were on our way, to which he responded with some rant about the parking warden not thinking this was very funny, and we were off – I was drowsy and being whipped around underground corridors in a wheelchair, we were rushing along the halls – I could see the door, I could feel the cold winter wind blowing toward us and we burst out onto the street – he wasn't there. How could he not be there? I called him – he was at the *other* loading dock – the one I was at was for ambulances and approved transport companies only. Fine, stay put, we were coming to him. Back into the hospital and the nurse was pushing my chair as fast as she could go, up an elevator and along an over-street passage, down another elevator and back through the winding, cement halls with flickering overhead lights and lost visitors wandering around – we didn't have time to give directions, we were on a mission!

We burst through this new set of doors into the frozen wind and I spotted our little blue SUV just a few yards away. Success! We had made it, and only two hours late! Paul leapt out of the car to collect me, his concern for me washing over his fury at my exceptionally poor timeliness – as he thanked the nurse, collected my notes, signed for me and helped me into the front seat of the car. I turned to wish the nurse a good night but she had already darted back into the warmth of the hospital, I couldn't really blame her. Paul put my seatbelt on, put my notes into the back of the car and climbed in himself, anxious to finally get going.

The car wouldn't start.

What? This is a great car! We've driven this thing all over Europe! We take great care of this thing! How could it not start?? He tried again. And again. And again. No dice, we weren't going anywhere. How could this happen? Ohhhhh. He'd been sitting idle waiting for me with my constant "five more minutes!" texts for nearly two hours. Gotcha. I laughed, but was silenced with "the look" which only a man can give when something has gone wrong with his car and it is clearly your fault. Like when I manage to somehow erase all of the Bluetooth data in the car system just by trying to change the radio station.

Well, I wasn't leaving that chair, I was too tired and drugged to really care anyway. This was up to him to sort out (I would have been useless at sorting it anyway) and I watched him google "road side assistance" as I drifted off to sleep.

Was woken up by angry husband – he wasn't supposed to let me fall asleep. The hospital staff had told him that I was to stay awake all the way back and there was *no* way I was going to slip into some sort of coma on his watch. Roadside assistance would be there within an hour and we just had to sit tight and wait. With no radio. And no heater. Even by Canadian standards this was already feeling pretty chilly. There was a blanket in the back we could use as a last resort but it wouldn't matter – roadside assistance would be here right away anyway. We waited in the frozen car, watching for a sign of any other vehicle that might be able to help us. A police car, a delivery van… anything. Nothing came. This area of hospital loading was deserted and dark. And eerily quiet. Paul refused to let me fall asleep just in case it was like anyone with a head injury – even though the drugs hadn't quite yet worn off, so we chatted, mostly about how cold we were and how ungodly long the roadside assistance was taking. We had been waiting for 45 minutes by that point, and my husband again called the roadside assistance number – they confirmed that a driver was on his way and would be there shortly, hang tight and stay warm. He threw his phone back into the middle console with a roar of frustration and I laughed, the absurdity of this situation was just too much. There we were, two Canadians freezing in a car with a dead battery, outside a hospital in which I'd just had minor surgery and was heavily drugged. Another hospital was expecting me, we were late and I still had a cannula in my arm (what is *with* those things?). And we had been waiting for roadside assistance for 57 minutes now – I couldn't help it, this was actually pretty bizarre and funny! Paul broke out into a laugh as we reveled at the situations we get ourselves into when, exactly 59 minutes after our first phone call, roadside assistance pulled up to the rescue.

Massive relief came over my husband's face as he popped the hood and leapt out of the car to greet the roadside assistance guy with jumper cables in hand. A battery pack was hooked up and then silence…nothing happened. My view from inside the car was obscured by the raised hood but I could hear them talking heatedly. Now they were arguing and Paul was insisting that they try once more, he didn't know what was wrong or why our battery was showing to be fully charged – he had surely drained the battery sitting outside for so long waiting for me! Paul came back into the car to give it a try – still nothing. Nothing at all. He moved out of the way for the roadside guy to have a go at starting the car – which he did, on the first try…

Once he tried to start the car in 'park' instead of 'drive', as my husband had been doing for the last hour.

I am the worst kind of person

I would generally classify myself as a pretty open, easy going and chilled out person when it comes to many things – a compassionate person in most cases as well (*most*). I would like to think that those that know me don't generally describe me as some sort of judgmental hatemonger but hey, not everyone can like you and I've come to accept that – in situations I can help. In others it's best just to blend back into the background and call a mulligan on it.

I was headed to the Stroke Clinic at Charing Cross hospital – giddy with the knowledge that this could very well be my last stroke clinic and keen to put the whole stroke ordeal behind me. I was so pumped I practically skipped there and totally didn't mind when a woman on the bus coughed all over me and then burped in my face. It's all good, I was heading for a formal discharge. Nothing could faze me today. I practically pranced up the hospital stairs and rocked up to one of their new automated patient check in kiosks (I'm not sure if this has actually helped to reduce staffing cost as the kiosks all have a staff member standing beside them waiting to walk anyone over 45 through the process. It can apparently be a very stressful experience – not least if you've just had a stroke, I'm sure.) and started checking in, only to find that I couldn't update my address on there and would have to line up at the regular desk now anyway. Fine.

The lineup was rather huge. Quite huge in fact, mostly full of old people that had burst into tears and given up on the automated kiosks, even with the helper, and have now sworn off touch screen technology altogether. That's fine, I wasn't in a rush – I was totally getting discharged! There's a commotion up front, a young guy making a lot of noise. As you do, I joined everyone else in peeking about in the hope of seeing some good line action only to realize that the gentleman had special needs, a helmet and a carer with him. Ah, I'm sure he's fine, best not to stare. A bit more time passes and a screech erupts from just behind me in the line and I jump, as do many others, turning in surprise to identify the source of the screech.

Behind me was a frazzled looking woman and her daughter of around eight years old who also seemed to have special needs and was in a specially formed wheelchair. The mother was restraining the girls' hands as the girl thrashed about – the mother then put headphones on the girl and set up a movie on an iPad for her, the thrashing stopped and all was calm again in the line. A young man meekly approached the girl's mother and told her that she was doing a wonderful job and that her patience and fortitude was an example to us all. The whole thing was very touching and quite warm and fuzzy to be a part of. Very lovely, but still, best not to stare.

The lined inched forward and the girl's wheelchair became positioned somewhat next to me rather than behind me and, having absolutely nothing else to do while I waited in line, I stole a glance at the girl's iPad to check out what she was watching.

This kid was watching the most absolutely freaking horrifying children's movie (?!?) I have ever, ever experienced. It had some sort of creepy skeletal animation similar to The Nightmare Before Christmas and she was still on the opening credits. I watched, glued to the screen and jaw slowly dropping in horror as a children's doll was undressed and then sliced apart in a methodical, serial killer type fashion. I recoiled in horror as the doll's eyes were pulled off, the woolen hair slowly torn from its head and its sewn mouth sliced open from end to end. What the hell kind of children's movie *was* this?!?! I couldn't look away. I shivered and folded my arms, my shoulders hunched up in disgust. A slit was made into the doll's side and the *stuffing was ripped out* and the empty cloth shell of a doll was then *hung on a meat hook* upside down. I stared with wide eyes and a horrified, disgusted look on my face. What the *hell* movie was this?!!?? This thing would give *me* nightmares and an eight year old is just chilling out watching this doll snuff movie?! Oh wait- the wheelchair moved violently to the left and right out of the line, jerking me back to reality. The mother stormed away throwing me the dirtiest look I'd ever seen back over her shoulder.

What was *that* for? That was weird. No matter, the line was inching forward again and I was nearly at the desk.

Except that everything was suddenly very quiet. And everyone was looking at me. They weren't nice looks, they were looking at me like I was the scum of the earth. What the hell? This was weird. Best to just look at the ground and not say anything. Did I have something on my shirt? Had I lost a tooth or something? I self-consciously wiped at my chin and felt around for food in my teeth. Something was up.

I got to the reception desk and even the receptionist was really cold to me, she would barely look me in the eye and her demeanor was just so rude – what was the…I followed her gaze back down the hall to the furious looking mother with her special needs daughter watching that horrible movie… oh God, no. Oh no. No no no no no. Did they think that I was reacting to her *daughter?!?* That I was staring and recoiling in horror at a child with special needs? In a *wheelchair*?!? As it dawned on me I looked around – they did. Oh no, even the mother thought I did. I looked back at the receptionist, helpless but desperate to clear my name – I was not a monster, I was just watching the kid's iPad like a creeper in line! Oh no, no no no no no. I did the only thing I could possibly think of and loudly, *desperately* declared to the receptionist:

"That kid has the creepiest movie I have ever seen on her iPad. I'm not going to sleep for a week!"

The receptionist warmed to me, a little, and I managed to squeak out my new address before slinking off to find a hole to crawl into and die. I don't think the other waiting patients bought my story and I sat there for nearly thirty minutes enduring the looks, stares and whispered admonishments until they were all replaced by a fresh wave of patients who hadn't witnessed my hideous social crime. I was the very worst type of human being. What could I do? Apologize to the mother? Explain myself? Go up and ask her what the *hell* her daughter was watching? I couldn't face the mother, I could barely face the other patients, and nearly jumped out of my skin at the sound of a wheelchair coming around the corner – eventually hiding out in the bathroom until the mother and her daughter had left. I was so embarrassed I could have cried

I am a terrible, terrible person. And I'm *still* not going to sleep for a good week.

It turns out it was the opening sequence to 'Coraline'. What the ever-loving crap. If I saw that in a theater I would have shat myself. I youtube'd it when I got home by searching for the keywords: "doll movie sequence creepy as f***" and it came right up, so clearly it's not just me.

What...the hell.

Am so glad I was discharged and never have to go back there again. But hey, yay for being discharged from the stroke clinic!

Chapter Five: The Side Effects can be Worse than the Disease

Side effects can often be almost worse than the disease itself. In about six months I went from a thin, well-adjusted yet near blind and violently arthritic woman to an obese hyped-up squirrel-like balding and infertile woman who would have mugged a homeless person for their pick of dumpster-diving culinary delights. And I was *still* near blind and violently arthritic.

Some things took getting used to. Like hair loss. I'd had long, soft blonde hair that suddenly came out in giant clumps in the shower. It now looked as though a blonde Yeti had been shaved and murdered in there. Even pre-empting the traumatizing hair loss by having my locks trimmed down to a pixie cut (which did *not* suit my swollen steroid face) made little difference to my husband's frequent complaints of me 'leaving a dead mouse-looking thing in the bathtub drain'.

Medications would bring me to the verge of narcolepsy in which I became *that* person on the tube – we all know the type. The one who falls asleep on a stranger's shoulder, snores loudly and then, realizing it is their stop, jumps up without warning and darts for the open doors of the train, smashing into them face first as they slide closed. I then spend the brief journey to the next station nursing my face *and* my pride, fearful of sitting down again lest the sudden narcolepsy and lemming-like door behavior take me again once more.

The nausea. Oh, the nausea. Debilitating waves mixed with my own 'projectile vomit paralysis' in which, when presented with the urge to heave, I simply cannot move. The most I can do is open my mouth and hope for the best. It's been like this ever since I can remember. As a teenager I once managed to hold in my nausea all way home from school – in a frantic rush I darted through the house and to the bathroom toilet, only to find our cat *inside* the sparkling white toilet bowl having a cool drink. I grabbed the cat around the middle and pulled, trying to get it out of the toilet so I could let loose my sick but the cat wasn't moving. She spread out all four paws under the seat and wedged herself in the bowl. It was coming. Panicked paralysis had set in. The thought of turning to the sink or bathtub didn't even cross my mind as my mouth opened and I covered the cat in a torrent of teenage sick.

I am now at the point that when my husband would notice that I had gone suddenly very still and very quiet – that would be his cue to grab a bucket and aim. I cannot bring myself to be sick into a toilet, either. Given what usually goes in there I just can't put my face that close to one unless it is freshly clean and absolutely spotless. For a while my husband kept the house well-armed with toilet brushes and bleach so that it was always in easy reach if need be, running to scrub the toilet if my skin color gave off hints of green. I once made it to the washroom by myself, desperately scrubbing away at the toilet when up it came – the toilet wasn't finished – and I threw up on the floor *beside* the toilet instead. Even on my husband's thirty-third birthday I had gotten him a loving and thoughtful gift of a golf club kit and a day out with the boys but ruined the delivery by launching projectile sick all over him in the middle of saying 'Happy Birthday'. He claims it was a birthday to remember and his favorite one so far. Sigh.

Some side effects are worse than others. Some creep up on us by surprise, like blood-thinners causing any cut I get to look like a violent crime scene. Some we hate with a passion and debate their worth – others we learn to live with. The steroid weight gain has been one of the hardest for me – if anything for just no longer recognizing the person in my mirror.

But hey. Better to be fat than dead.

Wait. More like, fat, bald, infertile, raging, weepy and nauseas than dead.

Maybe just better not to be dead.

Like Jabba the Hut in Drag

A rather charming and attractive side effect of prolonged steroid use is weight gain. No, not the type of steroids that pump you up and come with a lifetime supply of thongs and body oil – the *other* type of steroids. Weight gain, mood swings, insomnia, acne, diabetes, glaucoma, appetite monstrosity and inappropriate hair growth are common side effects of high dose steroids such as prednisolone, to name a few.

It has been a highly frustrating experience in that the side effects of chemotherapy drugs were hair loss on my head while the steroids put hair pretty much anywhere *but* on my head. My eyebrows bushed out like the Gruffalo and my nose hair grew to stick outside my nose. My nose hair grew so ridiculously fast that I would pluck a few in the morning and by mid-afternoon others were poking out and tickling my nose. I looked like I had developed some sort of tic I was scratching my nose so often – even more surprising was the discovery that my nose hair was now strangely multicolored and grew at a rather alarming rate for a woman.

The weight gain is an unbearable beast with steroids – an effect most patients of this drug experience. My pulmonologist warned me before starting that she had tried this drug once, just to see how bad the effects really were. This was a fairly thin, healthy vegetarian doctor – she told me that on the second night she woke up at three in the morning, snuck downstairs and cooked herself a full English breakfast. Sausages, eggs, beans, tomatoes, hash browns and toast with a glass of milk *and* a glass of orange juice. She was so ashamed of herself that she cleaned up all of the evidence and snuck back to bed – her husband never to know – and *still* woke up starving the next morning.

On steroids I would eat pretty much anything, any time. I was like a Tolkien hobbit with breakfast and 'secondsies' and then brunch. Even healthy food. Salad? Great! Pass me the bag and a fork! Apples? Two please! I'd have just eaten and my stomach would be burning – the fizz of acid audible when I opened my mouth. I would *obsess* about food – more than I had ever imagined was possible. It could be anything. Strawberries. Chocolate. Bananas. Spinach. Water. It was worse than any pregnancy craving I had ever experienced by far.

I once craved nachos – salted tortilla chips with shredded cheese and bbq sauce. Strange, and viciously unhealthy. But I *needed* them . I woke up in the morning having dreamt about nachos. My husband was still sleeping beside me – we had everything we needed in the kitchen to make them. The kids were sleeping – I could sneak downstairs and have nachos for breakfast and then clean it all up before anyone would be the wiser! But the dog – that stupid tap-dancing shihtsu would follow me and give me away. Not unless I picked him up and carried him with me the whole time though!

"Huarhuar!" I whispered. He looked up at me "Huarhuar!" I had his attention from his spot at the foot of our bed. "Come here buddy…" I whispered with hushed desperation. My stomach was growling and burning – my jaw stung as my mouth watered at the thought of breakfast nachos. I slowly got on all fours and crept down the bed and toward the dog, eager to grab him before he could jump down onto the hardwood floor with his clickity-clackity tap dancing nails – spinning as he always does in excitement. The dog was 12 years old! Why couldn't he just behave like an old dog and shuffle quietly around the house?

"Huarhuar… stay… come to mummy…" I slowly lowered my leg to the ground to get a good standing before grabbing the dog. My leg touched the ground and his ears perked up – we were going outside! Outside! *Outside*!

"Huarhuar no! Shhhhhh!!!!" I growled as he sprung off the bed like a deer and tap danced around my lowered leg – waking up my husband and stirring the kids in the next room.

Damn. Porridge for breakfast it would be.

Again.

Alright, fine. I shouldn't be eating nachos anyway. Terribly bad for me. Terribly. But I *could* have them for lunch. Instead of this stupid salad I made last night I could just go to a pub near the office and have nachos! I could go by myself – at around 10:30am so I would completely beat the lunch rush. Nobody would know! Nachos!

I did the smart thing and handed over all of my cash, bank and credit cards to my husband.

The entire hour long commute on the tube to work I thought about nachos. I didn't know why – I don't even *like* cheese. I just really, really wanted those nachos. I started to wonder who at work I could borrow money from – or could I have a business lunch by myself and use the company card? What if I borrowed some money, went to Tesco's, bought the stuff I needed and then microwaved myself some nachos at work on a paper towel plate? I could do that! Now, who to ask to borrow money from…

I refrained. Not very professional behavior when you're the boss.

I still couldn't stop thinking about those damn nachos though. Maybe I could go home early? Maybe I just should. I'm certainly not being very productive at work today anyway – can't stop thinking about stupid nachos. Alright, I'll go home at four-thirty then. May as well. Then I can at least justify having nachos for dinner or something.

By the time I had gotten home I had *completely* planned out my nacho extravaganza. I was going to walk in, say hi to the husband and kids, wash my hands and then make the nachos. I was going to use both the white cheddar and the red Leicester cheese and I was going to layer it and I was going to put on chili powder and … what do you mean dinner is ready? *What do you mean soup?!*

By the end of the day I found that the only way to curb my ravenous craving for nachos was to empty the entire contents of the tortilla chip bag into the bin so I wouldn't be tempted to dig it out later. The act nearly had me in tears, but it had to be done. This level of craving wasn't normal and I couldn't give in to it.

I wonder if you can make nachos with toast?

Do muumuus come in designer labels?

Even with my stalwart rejection of obsessive food cravings my weight quickly reached a level that was well out of control. I had gained 80lbs in a year. A single year! Steroids pile on weight like you wouldn't believe, but not just from eating. It changes the way that your body processes your food, it causes extreme water retention and redistributes weight to weird areas, giving you Cushingoid or Cushing's Syndrome, a lovely condition in which you get a round "moon face", a fat hunchback "buffalo hump" and a nice round belly. Like an egg with stick legs.

I had been eating what I thought to be a very healthy diet in an effort to stop this rapid weight gain. I was a vegetarian. I stopped eating dairy products. I stopped eating processed foods and went on a 'real food' diet in which if my great grandmother wouldn't recognize it as food I wouldn't eat it. I cooked everything from scratch with fresh, wholesome ingredients. I made my own organic smoothies packed with fruit and vegetables. I drank only pure organic juice or water. I cut pineapples and learned to slice a mango from youtube. Nothing was working – I would get another steroid infusion in hospital and gain 10lbs that week – every single time. It was awful.

I hadn't quite realized how bad it had gotten until I went for a bone density scan at the hospital and was told that I couldn't have the scan, I was over the weight limit by 2kg and might break the table.

I remember nodding politely and putting my clothes back on, quietly containing any reaction until I had found a quiet hospital stairwell to cry in. I called my husband from the stairwell and told him that I should give up and buy a fat-scooter – did he think they came in 'double wide'?

How could this be happening to me? I cooked fresh food! No oil! I wasn't just getting my five a day, I was getting fifteen! I had cut out wheat, dairy, eggs, sugar and processed foods. How was this happening?

My diet had a distinct lack of Whoppers, chips, crisps, chocolate, pop, lattes, pizza and KFC. I *looked* like I spent my days lying around in a floral muumuu eating takeout pizza and watching cheap daytime television riddled with personal injury lawyer commercials with the curtains drawn. This wasn't me! I wanted to write "I'm a vegan!" on a t-shirt but was worried that it would look more like I'd eaten a vegan than actually was one.

As I walked back to my waiting husband and children in the hospital parking lot I wondered what life would be like as a bulimic fruitarian.

The Jeans Incident

There was certainly an adjustment period – medications and side effects alone provided an incredible amount of entertainment. Just the other day I was all happy because I had bought a new pair of jeans and as I put them on I realized that they were too big. Although very comfy, I had to keep hiking them up a bit at the waist. No worries, they look better than my too-tight jeans and this means I must be losing weight. I'm smaller than I thought, how great!

So I wore them to work and as the day went on they somehow got bigger. Or I got smaller. One of the two. Possibly a combination of both. By about noon I was spending less time on work and more time looking at belts on Amazon. My boss asked me to a meeting at a posh Barrister's office with our £500 an hour lawyers and into a taxi we went, him getting in like a normal person and me trying to hide the fact that both hands were jammed into my pockets not because they were cold but because that was the only reasonably inconspicuous way to hold my pants up at that point. Getting out of the taxi was much worse, trying to grip my bag with one hand and my jeans with the other whilst bending over to lurch out of a black cab with any grace whatsoever- it wasn't pretty but he wasn't looking.

We had arrived downtown London at a beautiful old courthouse building in the sweltering heat, squinting up at the sun and waiting for our team of barristers to find us outside. They arrived from their air conditioned offices with effortless grace and expensive suits, tall black heels and perfectly knotted chignons. Niceties were exchanged as I abandoned my oversized bag on my shoulder in favor of gripping my now much too large jeans to my body, freeing one hand for customary handshakes and air kisses (which as a Canadian woman

I still don't quite get and end up *actually* kissing someone half the time. Very awkward). Our little troupe entered the tiny doorway of the old, tall courthouse building and started up a narrow, thickly carpeted staircase in a silent conga-line of professionalism and expense, making small talk about our case and light comments about the unusually warm summer.

And what do I do?

I trip and fall down the stairs - and as I got up and braced myself against a wall my jeans completely fell down. To the floor. Around my ankles and just like a cartoon, my bare legs boldly displayed across the stair case in a flash of bright sweaty whiteness.

I stood there in horror, grasping at my legs and feeling only bare skin. They've all turned around to look and the lawyer behind me is having an internal battle of either lunging to help me or turning away and averting his eyes. I reached for my jeans with one hand while gripping the bannister with the other for fear of plummeting down again and was in such an awkward position that my jeans wouldn't slide all the way back up, they're hovering now around my thighs, stuck to my damp skin. They've tasted freedom and they weren't going back on without a fight.

So I'm standing there in a panic desperately clutching at my jeans and trying to yank them back up (I've completely abandoned my bag at this point and another lawyer ran to get it) while my boss is looking at me with a mix of concern and sheer disbelief - the three lawyers were all fussing over me asking if I'm okay and I'm trying as best as possible to regain my composure and assure them that I'm fine, nothing to see here! A couple of grunts and two handed jump-thrusts and my jeans are firmly back up around my waist, my breathing returns to somewhat normal and we continue up the stairs - and as we do, every time we came to a slight dip in the next floor all four of them turned to me and reminded me to "be careful!"

Yep. Saw it, thanks. For like, three more flights of stairs.

We all go on all pretending as though this didn't just happen and continue on to sit around a posh conference table talking about a very serious matter concerning international child protection and kidnapping laws and, complete moron that I am, I start giggling. It is absolutely horrifying but I cannot stop. I'm breaking into chuckles and sniggers and it's going round and round in my head - are they thinking about it too? Are they waiting for me to leave so they can all laugh about it? Should I tell them that I'm diseased? Tell them that my medication causes rapid daily weight loss and gain? Play the sympathy card? Oh God, they're all thinking about it. I can totally tell.

Someone asked me what it was I found so funny and I went on a quick cover-up about "the irony of the case was just very amusing" Oh my God it was horrible. And then, when I thought I had composed myself over further serious discussions, the imagery popped back into my head and, I kid you not, I let out a Scooby Doo giggle. It sounded EXACTLY like Scooby Doo. You know the one - *hee HEE hee hee hee*.

It's a wonder some days how I am still employed.

Offensive Eggs

I'd recently taken a business trip to Northern England with some colleagues to meet with a University partner for an event. I like to pack light and as a large woman it can be somewhat difficult to dress very nicely. Having become accustomed to my size varying greatly at any point in a day as a nice additional medication side effect (hence the jeans incident earlier) I opted for comfort over style and wore nice yet comfortable dark jeans with a loose top that showed what was now my best feature – my steroid cleavage.

Which was fine, until I was at breakfast with my colleagues and I dropped a great splotch of scrambled egg off my fork on the way to my mouth – and it landed directly in my cleavage. It was half in and half out – jiggling for all to see as my two male work colleagues stared openly at my egg cleavage before quickly looking away and pretending not to have seen.

What could I do? I couldn't just reach in and dig it out! I picked up a napkin and pretended to dab at my shirt, dislodging half of the egg chunk and now grasping it in my hand. The other half was still in there. There was really no way to deal with this in a lady-like manner, but I wasn't going to go digging around in there for it at the table. Maybe I could wiggle my top a bit and it would come out the bottom, I could then get it out by reaching around under the table and out of sight.

I skooched my chair closer to the table and bent forward slightly, assuming I looked inconspicuous but my eyes were wide like a deer in headlights. I shook the shirt. Nothing. "It's certainly warm in here." I remarked openly, to no one. They weren't looking. The topic of football had come up and they were engaged in a heated debate about some cup I'd never heard of. Thank God. I shook my shirt again. A bit of slimy jiggling, but still no movement. This wasn't working. I would have to finish my breakfast like it didn't happen and then just be the last to leave the table. Make up some excuse to stay behind and deal with it then, no worries.

Except that I had completely forgotten about it by the end of the meal and got up with my colleagues, pushing away from the table and heading off back to our rooms together to collect our bags. We made small talk as we entered the elevator in a semi-circle of conversation about the upcoming event preparation that still needed to be done when suddenly all was silent as the three of us stared at the ground;

The remaining egg had fallen out of my top and bounced off of the shoe of our Director of Academic Development. There it was, the offending chunk of scrambled cleavage egg, there on the floor staring up at us.

There's just not much you can say in a situation like

that.

Damn steroids.

You've got to do things slowly – or you just look like a jerk.

Apparently you cannot just 'stop' taking steroids and must wean off them very slowly as you will go into adrenal shock and your body will essentially shut down. My recent experience with adrenal shock after having merely forgotten a morning dosage has now reinforced this doctrine in my mind – something I am not eager to experience again. Weaning off these things, however, is no easy feat on its own. A person weaning off many types of medication, including steroids, may go through symptoms of drug withdrawal ranging from pain and a rise in symptoms to mania and wild mood shifts. Temporary personality changes, even. It's a pretty wild ride.

It was officially day seven of reduced steroids. My insatiable rage hunger seemed to have subsided slightly, and I was no longer tempted to root through rubbish bins like a homeless person looking for things to eat. I'm viewing this as a positive. However, other problems are coming back. Also, my right eye hurts and makes a squishing sound when I blink - and I have the emotional stability of a suicide bomber.

Am tempted to inform the doctors, but am also keen to avoid another round of captivity and macaroni and cheese suspiciously lacking in macaroni.

Decisions, decisions.

I am, however, a complete jerk of a person some days-
even more so with these steroid mood swings of panic
and rage. I stopped by the supermarket on the way
home from work to pick up some things for dinner and
my lunches for the week - managed, for the first time
ever, to shop *only* in the vegetable aisle. Oh yes, nine
quid worth of green leafy vegetables, red cherry
tomatoes, bright orange carrots and deep green
avocados. Nom nom nom. Upon finishing my shop I
was faced with the dilemma of a short, near non-
existent queue at the self-checkout or a reasonably long
queue at the regular check out. My inner jerk-face self
proceeded to the regular checkout because really, why
do such a great and healthy shop if there's nobody to
see it!?!

So there I was, lining up my vegetables in an elaborate
display of judgment and condescension on the conveyer
belt between other people's bounty full of chocolate
bars, frozen pizza and white bread. My little oasis of
"in-your-face" healthfulness and a testament to a "holier
than thou" iron will of diet determination, standing tall
and proud as a peacock as I watched others eye up my
stash with puzzlement and defeat.

My body language screamed "look at this, you weak
slaves to consumerism and processed sugar! Look at all
of this green! Ha! The bread aisle temptress did not stay
me from my list like it did you! I breezed by the
reduced double chocolate chunk muffins and scoffed at

142

the sweets aisle with disdain! Ha! I did not even fall for the sneaky check-out gum! Ha ha ha ha ha ha!"

I looked to my left at the woman in front of me with her few vegetables and low-fat, no-carb, no-sugar yogurt. Ha! I have NO yogurt. I win! (Oooh, half price Doritos! Damn it! No!) I managed to leave the supermarket with my two bags full of wholesome, healthful goodness and an unreasonable amount of pride in myself - and no Doritos! Ha! I'd won the supermarket check-out judgment contest today! I won! I won!

I am a complete jerk, but after a day of reading online about steroid weight gain and obsessing about how to control it it's really the little things in life that get you through and give you a reason to laugh at yourself.

Plus, my husband has to go back to the store later. He can pick up Doritos then.

Any change in steroids will give me insomnia and affect my mood. I get frazzled by very ordinary situations and overwhelmed by things like my toothbrush. I've not yet learned to stay at home during these changes, but I should.

Things that shouldn't be stressful become suddenly and completely overwhelming, like the incredibly stressful situation of having to bag my own groceries at Sainsbury's. It's a scramble of epic proportions in which I always get my debit card out first before the conveyer belt has even started to move, panic about where to put my card (do I put it back in my purse and risk the Great Purse Scramble of Desperation in which the card will surely secure itself to an obscure yet effective hiding place while I fumble around like a bear in oven mitts and apologize profusely to the impatient line up accumulating behind me?!?) and then resign myself to holding my debit card (unnecessarily and prematurely) between my teeth throughout the entire bagging process.

You then dart to the bagging area / time trial zone to do frantic battle with those bloody orange plastic bags that *will not* come apart and open properly – all the while becoming quickly buried in your various purchases as the cashier maliciously slides the items toward you faster and faster with absolutely no regard to the careful pre-packing preparations you had made while lining them up. Milk is somehow followed by eggs and delicate cupcakes as you try, Tetris style, to stack them in the clingy bags in the hope that you will at least have *some* usable eggs left when you get home, only to be slammed with an onslaught of orange juice cartons and an eight pack of yogurt. The yogurt explodes but you cannot stop, though your thoughts are screaming "Abort! Abort!" The cashier cares not for the struggles of the amateur grocery-bagger and everyone in the line is glaring at you, willing you to just bag up your food and go – all the while judging your food choices from the small pile of Kettle Chips to the ready-made Trifles. You flamboyantly reach for and show off your head of broccoli and carton of soy milk to the masses, desperate to convince these strangers that your diet is really very healthy and you're surely just picking up these Krispy Kremes for someone else. It's not like you can even say anything to them, as you've still got a debit card wedged in between your teeth.

By then I just want to get out of there. I don't care if I've left a bag on the floor. I don't care how much it cost. Half the time I don't even look. I pay, grab what I can and slink out the door, exhausted and sweating, shrouded in shame at my bagging failure. I won't even *attempt* the self-check-out.

And surely, once I get home my husband takes all of eight seconds to announce that I had forgotten the cheese and I burst into tears. I'm given a hug, a warm cup of tea and resolve myself to online grocery shop from now on.

Until the next time we need cheese.

Putting the 'fun' in bodily functions

Most people that have ever spent much time in a hospital understand that the various medications you take can sort of slow things down in the bodily function department. Things can slow to a grinding halt – resorting to desperate remedies such as more medication to counteract the *other* medication, desperate prayer to non-descript deities and, in particularly hopeless situations, extreme medical intervention.

This is how I once found myself with a doctor giving me an enema at four in the morning on my living room couch shortly after having had my twins.

It just happens.

I'd started working with a private dietician for help in counteracting my Cushing's syndrome steroid weight – which had gotten very extreme by that point. I'd found, however, that my new restrictive diet kind of blocked things up. I wasn't expecting this at all – surely drinking so much water and the sheer amount of beans in my diet would have sorted this issue out. No, she said. We would need to help this along. She prescribed a mild laxative drink, to be taken once in the morning and once in the evening. Just to help things along.

"What if they helped things along *too* much?"

She told me not to worry about it, this was just mild. She has another regular patient with severe digestive issues, who will undoubtedly go running to the washroom only moment after trying any new food. She once encouraged him to try eating grapes – which he did. He apparently loved them and, experiencing no ill effect, ate the entire bunch before getting on the London underground to go to work.

People are apparently *not* terribly sympathetic when a man in a suit completely soils himself on the tube. He had no choice but to stay firmly in his seat until the train had reached its final stop at the end of the line, at which point he could exit in relative solitude to clean himself up and make his way home.

Laughing at her story I vowed to take the laxative without fear and report back the next week. Over the next few days my predicament became painful to the point that I started to genuinely wonder if things could possibly come back up the other way and googling whether or not a person could actually die from constipation. I was taking the laxative but there was no change. I returned to the box – reading that an adult can safely take up to six packets a day. Why not? I was very desperate at this point – it was a mild prescription anyway.

I took a packet that evening with dinner. Then another with my evening meds just before bed. Nothing. A third packet in the morning with breakfast and headed off to work. Still nothing. A fourth packet as a mid-morning snack and a fifth over lunch. Still nothing! I was trying yoga positions and deep breathing exercises. Still nothing. A sixth packet during afternoon tea. This was getting serious – perhaps I would call the out of hours clinic when I got home. I couldn't believe that I had taken all those packets and still nothing was happening.

I'd been on the tube for about 20 minutes when I started to feel a bit ill. Unusually warm and flushed. Thankfully I was already sitting down but the train was still rather packed with rush-hour commuters – none of them looked overly warm or uncomfortable. I felt my forehead and was surprised to feel my cold and clammy skin. I was sweating, too. An immense grumble erupted from my lower intestines – audible throughout the train. I joined the others in looking around for the source of the sound so as not to draw attention to myself, though I was the only one sat there sweating and grimacing in pain. My guts felt as though they were twisting into a knot. Oh God, not here. Not now. No no no no no.

I looked up at the tube map – we'd just passed white city and I had seven more stops to go. I just had to make it home.

I have a massive fear of public washrooms. After having lived in rural China for so long I had encountered public washrooms so horrifying that I had opted to go *behind* the washroom rather than in it. I've also got an experience with a Chinese hospital urinal that traumatized me for life, but that is a story for another day. Train station washrooms, actually – nearly *any* public washroom, is an absolute last resort for me. At my office I only use one bathroom and have arranged the janitor to clean it a minimum of three times a day. I've got issues, I'm cool with that. In a public washroom I am careful not to touch anything and if I cannot hover over the seat I layer it in toilet paper to prevent any unfortunate public toilet seat contact. Best to just avoid at all costs, really.

Train station bathrooms in London are a little less vile, but mostly because you have to pay 20 pence to use them. My theory is that this is a great act of cruelty on behalf of Transport for London, as nobody keeps 20 pence coins on them and any person desperate enough to use a train station washroom will clearly not be organized and clear-headed enough to calmly *find* their 20 pence coin – resulting in a load of people dancing around outside these locked washrooms frantically digging around in purses and pockets, begging perfect strangers for change and soiling themselves just outside the door. With the amount of cameras that TFL has within their stations I am sure that this provides much entertainment. I still think it's cruel.

Five more stops and I was already clenching my cheeks together, thinking back to my dietician's story about the man on a train in a suit. This was getting severe. I searched my bag and pockets – no 20 pence piece. Not a single coin at all to be found and even if I had, most stations don't even have washrooms! This would be a helpful thing to have on the tube diagrams. They show you where there is step-free access at which stations but not those with public washrooms. Sheer cruelty.

Another rumble. Oh god, things were starting to really move around in there. I was in a full cold sweat now – my hands were shaking. This was going to happen. I pulled out my phone to text my husband:

"Laxative emergency. Won't make it home if walk. Bring car to station. And towels."

"Can't. Picking up pizza with kids. Won't be home for 20 min. Can you wait at station?"

"Am about to have train incident. Will not make it home"

"Am definitely not picking you up in the car then."

By now I was writhing around in the seat trying to inconspicuously relieve some noxious pressure (don't judge, I thought I was dying!). People were starting to notice and backed away, opting to stand rather than to sit in a seat anywhere near me. I was sweating profusely by then – eyes glued to the tube map above and counting the stations until I could get home. Hanger Lane – that's a large station, would they have a washroom? Even a staff washroom? Could I possibly beg and persuade my way in to a TFL staff washroom? Pretend I was pregnant? The doors had already closed – on to Perivale. No *way* was I getting out at Perivale to look for a washroom.

This had gone beyond desperate as I held everything in as best as I could, leaning to the side to relieve pressure in a nonchalant "I'm just leaning here because I'm so relaxed" expression that was fooling no one. Another rumble and I nearly lost control. Sounds were erupting from my stomach that I'd never before experienced – loud, violent eruptions like vaguely muffled trumpets of shame. I was perched on the edge of my seat now, having decided that if Greenford looked like a relatively abandoned outdoor station I was going to make a run for it and let loose in the nearest foliage I could find. I nearly screamed out in anguish at the sight of some sort of school trip hanging around on the platform – foiling my opportunity – yet I managed to contain myself, gripping the blue cloth bench seat of the train as I strained to control my bowels. I cursed the dietician. I cursed the pharmacy – how could this stuff not come with some kind of red warning label? I vowed to never take anything like this again as we arrived at Northolt –

only one more stop, to find *more* people on the platform and no hope for a private explosion in a dark area of the platform.

A sudden thought occurred to me – my stop was next, but could I stand up? What was going to happen when I added *gravity* into this mix? Would I be able to keep it together? Do I just run off the train determined to not look back, heading for home in shame and humiliation? Did I have any other choice? This might just happen and no amount of willpower was going to make any sort of difference. I was in agony – sheer, audible agony. Staying on the train was just not an option – I would have to make a run for it.

The tube slowed into the station and I prepared myself with one foot pressed vertically against the bench base like a sprint runner, ready to dash out the nearest double door before whatever happened would have the chance to exit through the leg of my jeans. I was ready, this was going to be quick. God help anyone that got in my way. The buzzer sounded like a starting gun in that moment as the doors opened and I was up and out before they had fully slid to the side, running away from the train and down the stairs like my life depended on it. Diseased or not I bounded down those stairs and to the ticket gate faster than I'd ever gone before, all while stood tall and perfectly erect – which is what happens when you are clenching your bottom tightly enough to make a diamond.

I was out, into the open air! Into the dark! On automatic pilot I began to speed-walk the ten minute journey

home, I was going to make it! Another violent rumble
let loose from below and I was tempted to allow
another small release of noxious pressure but terrified
that I would gamble and lose. I was *not* going to make
it home, there was just no way. I came to the abandoned
pizza shop with a dark and relatively secluded parking
lot. The type typically reserved for drug deals and that
had a suspicious looking mattress in the back corner. I
considered the rubbish strewn small bush of foliage at
the back of the darkened lot as a spot to let loose but
hesitated at the thought of what worse I might find back
there.

My entire body was trembling and I was beginning to
feel faint as I turned and sprinted for the nearby
Sainsbury's, a horrifying public washroom. I had
surpassed desperation and it was closer than my home –
and even if I somehow made it home there was no
guarantee I would make it up the carpeted stairs to the
washroom. I burst through the doors and into the bright
overhead lights of the Sainsbury's, searching all signs
for directions to the washroom yet finding none.
Feeling guilty and not wanting to appear as someone
who had come in solely to take advantage of their
washroom facilities I penguin-shuffled over to the
baskets to collect one, filled it with magazines and a
bouquet of flowers and then ran to the security desk for
directions to the customer washrooms. I looked like a
maniac running down the aisles and darting past
pensioners that seemed determined to get in my way.
The washroom was in sight and I ran in, flinging my
blue basket of magazines and flowers toward a nearby
bench with wild abandon as I burst into the loo –

thrilled at finding it empty and relatively clean. I didn't even have time to layer the seat in toilet paper squares. What followed were a series of sounds and events typical only of a Mexican roadside truck-stop and pathetic texts to my husband that I would from then on be living in the Sainsbury's washroom, too humiliated to ever leave, and how shall we set up visitation for the children?

I've since requested a more natural and less violent range of relief from my dietician. Like grapes or Indian curry. Anything, *anything* but those stupid little packets of lies and disaster.

Don't Judge Me Doritos

My husband, bless him, tries to be helpful. This is much appreciated during hospital stays as he will bring daily bits of home comforts like clean clothes, new books, proper vegetables and homemade fruit salads to counteract my constant hospital diet of macaroni and cheese suspiciously lacking in macaroni. I was trying to stick to healthy and healthful food – anything that might help my body repair itself and get better.

So when he brought me an external hard drive full of new movies, a family bag of Doritos and some salsa I was touched by his kind gesture of essentially giving me a hospital 'movie night' but hid it all under my bed so it would be 'out of sight out of mind'. The steroid infusions were already piling on weight and giving me the most bizarre and obsessive cravings I'd ever imagined. I simply *couldn't* subject my body to

153

devouring a family sized bag of Doritos and salsa. Well, I shouldn't.

It probably wouldn't be a good idea.

The problem is that these drugs also give a person insomnia. The incessant noise and light of a hospital ward doesn't help much either, but I suddenly found myself wide awake at five in the morning and absolutely starving.

The kitchen wasn't open. The cafeteria wasn't open and even if it was I wasn't able to make it there with how many wires I had connecting me to the wall anyway. There was no way I was going to be able to fall back asleep so I reached over, fumbling in the dark, to find my laptop and the external hard drive beside the bed. My hand brushed against something crinkly... the Doritos! No, I couldn't. Not at five o'clock in the morning. *Completely* inappropriate.

I turned on Battleship, preparing to be engrossed in a terrible, terrible movie. The type in which you essentially remove your brain, pop it onto the shelf for a couple of hours and enjoy. Which I did, but I couldn't stop thinking about those Doritos.

I was watching a movie. Isn't that what snacks are for? The steroids were messing with my internal clock – my body probably thought that it was nighttime anyway, the perfect time for some snacks and a movie. What could it hurt? I was *so* hungry. I looked around the ward – everyone else was sleeping. I could pull the curtain and eat a couple of Doritos and nobody would be the wiser. Nobody would have to know. Like a ninja I unfolded my long legs and crept out of bed, gently and silently pulling the curtain around my little hospital campsite – always on the wide-eyed lookout for any one of the stern nurses that might suss out what I was up to.

Alone and enclosed in the privacy of my blue paper curtains I curled back up on the bed with glee, clutching my laptop, Doritos and salsa – my forbidden treasure. Nobody had to know. Nobody would ever know. I could hide the evidence before proper morning arrived – right after the movie.

So I settled and tucked in, so conscious of being found out that I was letting each Dorito chip soften in my mouth by sucking on it until I could crunch down without being too noisy. It was delicious. It was satisfying. It was so, so sinful. So wrong, but so good as I sat perched on my hospital bed watching a movie with my headphones on. I was like a twitchy squirrel eating a nut, not realizing after a while just how loud my chip crunching and salsa-sucking noises actually were –

Until a nurse threw back the curtain and stared as I screamed in alarm "DON'T JUDGE ME!!!" and threw the half-eaten bag of nachos back under the bed. (which she then confiscated). I clutched my chest trying to take calming breaths as the woman had scared me half to death, as I had her. Maybe she didn't see?

It was too late – I was covered in crumbs and salsa. I'd

clearly been exposed as an early morning crisp-and-salsa-muncher and labeled a "problem patient".

There's just no recovering from something like that.

Blue Badge Fun

Although I'd applied for one, there was a distinct sense of disappointment and fear upon receiving my 'Blue Badge' (a disabled parking pass) in the post.

On one hand, yay! I can now park wherever I want whenever I want. Kind of like a drunken schizophrenic with a license and a mission. Half on the sidewalk? Who cares! As long as it's only for three hours! On the lawn of Parliament? Middle of the fountain at Trafalgar Square? Why not!

On the other hand, well, yay for being officially "disabled"? This was something I could no longer hide from, that my preferred coping mechanism of straight up denial couldn't hide. Evidence of just how bad this was, how much my life had changed – was in my hand.

My doctor really pushed me to apply - although she told me it was near impossible to get one of these. She's seen people with terminal cancer and one leg be refused. Me though? They didn't even ask for more evidence aside from the initial letter I had sent. They just looked up my NHS record and thought "Holy hell, this woman is still *alive*?!?! And *working*?!?! Nutter!" and then signed off. I'm almost surprised my approval letter didn't come with a condolence card and a muffin basket.

I don't actually *need* it. Well, most of the time I don't, so I do only use it when absolutely necessary. The biggest plus being that my husband can now actually park outside the A&E entrance for my next stroke instead of pulling up and just rolling me out of the car. On treatment weeks it is very nice to have as I cannot walk far without draping myself over my children's pushchair for support and there have been more than a few times where I've had to sit down on the ground in a parking lot to catch my breath. For a woman that usually goes hiking every weekend this is extreme – and I need to get back to the safety of my car quite quickly (not that I drive- not able to any more).

My husband is more self-conscious about using the blue badge – and will only let me use it when I really, really need to. After all, disabled spaces are for disabled people – not just part time disabled people like me. There is a common perception of disabled people and just who is 'disabled enough' to use those spaces. I once saw a person pull up into a disabled parking space in a red Ferrari and noticed the people staring with disapproval. Even I was staring with disapproval – until he got out of the car using walking sticks and struggled his way across the walkway. Disabled parking space users must drive wheelchair adapted vans, obviously. Never would they drive a Ferrari, surely!

We once won a disabled parking space outside of a shopping center around Christmas after an epic experience in 'predatory parking'. I'd just had a treatment and, although very weak, was determined to do a bit of last minute stocking stuffer gathering at Boots, with my husband there to lean on and help me through. I guess I didn't look disabled enough as a family walking by made a snide comment about how "did I not see that we had parked in a disabled stall – it's not just there for lazy shopping." That stung.

I stopped and looked straight at the woman and told her that just because she couldn't see my disability that doesn't mean that she would possibly want what I've got.

Not to say that I couldn't understand her point of view – I certainly used to think the same. Though it made my husband a little bit more self-conscious about using the badge – we once parked outside a Tesco in the disabled stall. As we got out of the car people were staring, trying to gauge which of us was disabled and if it was worthy of that parking spot. I could see my husband squirming uncomfortably so to make him even *more* uncomfortable I affected a dramatic limp – limping all the way from the car to the store doors. He told me that I'd made my point, could I stop now? Wait, never mind – keep up the limp! Those same people are behind us!

So I limped, for no reason other than pride, around the vegetable isle trying to 'lose' this couple behind us. We couldn't shake them! They too were following our typical supermarket progression route. We tried to ditch them between laundry detergent and pet food – turns out they had a cat too. I continued to limp around the store, terrified that I would suddenly look like the ending scene of 'The Usual Suspects' going from a limp to walking normally around the supermarket.

A parking spot was so not worth it.

Chapter Six: Going Private

Too Posh for Signage

Walking into a private hospital in London is like walking into a hotel. A concierge stands outside to greet patients as they arrive and the reception desk staff are smartly dressed and attentive – would I like a fresh croissant on my way in? The halls are carpeted and the walls decorated with proper art, distinctly un-hospital like. Where was the signage? The rampant health and safety gone mad? Where were the colored lines painted along the floor directing you to where you need to go, or the hanging signs at each junction directing people to washrooms, elevators and the nearest fire extinguisher station? They simply weren't there – the patients of this hospital clearly either knew where they were going or were directed by the concierge upon entry.

This place was clearly far too posh for signage.

Which didn't quite work out well for me when one morning I was very late and running through the hospital like a madwoman, my doctor on the phone asking me if I was still coming. I assured her that I was just downstairs, actually, masking my frantic panting from the dash down the hall and through twisted corridors of an old building clearly expanded through randomized extensions. I would be right up, hang on!

And this is how I chased a man straight into the handicapped washroom like some sort of psychotic mental ward escapee.

I'd been running around this hospital without signage searching for the stairs when just ahead of me I saw another person running, a man – clearly he was also late and searching for the stairs but he seemed to know where he was going. So I followed him, still running, as you do. He looked back at me and slowed to a speed walk, so I slowed to a speed walk just behind him. He looked back at me again and picked up the pace, as did I. In hindsight it *may* have looked as though I was chasing him.

The man suddenly veered to the left and pushed through a large wooden door, making to close it behind him but I pushed through, I was in a hurry too! What was wrong with this guy? He screamed, actually screamed and shouted at me to get out and leave him alone – and then I realized that I was standing with him inside a handicapped washroom. I had chased a man down a hall and into a handicapped bathroom, like some kind of crazed mugger. I opened my mouth to… what, apologize? Stammer out an explanation? The only thing that burst out of my mouth was "Damn! Where are the stairs?!" as he shoved me out of the washroom and locked the door.

I really must pay more attention to my surroundings.

Going Private – or, debt, spiraling paranoia and Chinese slavery

As a kid growing up in Canada private versus public health care was not even on my radar. To me, I always got the care I needed, when I needed it and never had a reason to complain about the healthcare system. I liked Jell-O and hospitals had lots of it, what else was there to know?

You hear a lot of arguments, often quite misguided, coming out of the States about the horrors of nationalized health care such as Canada's – with our apparent cancer death panels and 12 year waiting periods for an MRI. I never had this problem, and it certainly wasn't from a lack of experience. By the time I left Canada at the tender (but infinitely wise and mature) age of 21 years old I had broken nearly all of my fingers and toes, an ankle, wrists, arms, ribs, a shoulder… my nose a few times…

And no, I was not a semi-professional boxer, wild bear wrangler or the personal assistant to a former child star. I was just accident prone and active. (I once broke my arm getting it on with my then boyfriend (now husband) in the shower. That was a fun one to explain at the hospital) That, and again, stuff just sort of *happened* to me. It always has.

I moved to China and, being the way I am, got a very good view over six years of the public healthcare system in China as well as the incredible affordability of those without proper coverage. Aside from a couple of incidents here and there (okay, quite a few doozies) I was quite content with the quality and speed of care there. As such, even as an expat in China for far longer than most I never felt the urge to purchase private insurance or to visit a private doctor or hospital. What was good enough for three billion others was more than good enough for me. Plus, each visit was an absolute adventure – how could I pass that up?

I once had an incident in Hong Kong and, although the care was phenomenal, to this day I don't recall having ever given so much as my name let alone any payment for that care, and wonder if I shoplifted emergency care. If anything, the most frightening healthcare experience I've had to date would have been in the States over the sheer cost of emergency care and the associated financial horror stories that this entails when I was hit by lightning in my late teens.

Here in the United Kingdom I've been nothing if not thoroughly impressed and elated with the care I have received on the public health system. My doctors and specialists are fantastic, the hospitals are efficient yet pleasant and I've never before felt frustration at having to wait for a test, procedure or result.

Until I had a miracle drug dangled in front of me like a life raft to a drowning rat.

The Great Brad Pitt (MD)

So I guess it is really only natural for people when diagnosed with a disease of any sort, be it diabetes, sarcoidosis or rampant hypochondria – to become almost overly knowledgeable about their condition. I certainly have – from the desperate nights alone in the hospital with nothing to do but incessantly google my condition on my iPhone – at one point all of my bed's electrical sockets were full and a nurse found me and my IV pole curled up to an electrical socket with my phone and power cord at three am on the floor in a dark hallway. I was a woman obsessed.

I read online medical journals. I read questions that had come up on yahoo and their associated strange, nonsensical answers. I read tabloid and newspaper articles about Bernie Mac and Michael Clarke Duncan, both having died from complications involving Sarcoidosis.

Confusingly, I seemed to have a disease that kills famous black men. Being neither famous nor a black man you'd think that this would make me feel somewhat better.

It didn't.

I found an online forum for those with Sarcoidosis and joined – excited to have found other people like me. I think that this perhaps scared me the very most (someone lost their nose to sarc. Their *nose!*) and more than a few people on the forum have passed away from complications due to their condition. These are just the ones that we've heard about – with close friends also on the site that are able to pass this news on. Many just disappear altogether and you can really just hope for the best – that they got better and stopped posting or their laptop exploded and took out half of their living room and they've sworn off ever touching a computer again, hence their sudden disappearance. Anything but 'sarc got 'em'.

The forum itself is often a depressing place full of messages of fear, confusion, frustration and the desperation of those reaching out in the hopes of finding someone, anyone, that has also experienced this and the symptoms unique to all of us with this disease that are often so impossible to explain. However, I have also found it to be a wealth of knowledge and experience from which to draw on and arm myself while obediently visiting specialist after specialist – all of them with different ideas and plans for my care.

The doctors gave me high-dose steroids (again, not the HULK SMASH fun kind. The bad kind) and told me to "watch my weight and mood" on them. The forum taught me what the steroids would really do to me. The doctors put me on methotrexate injections, telling me that "you might feel a bit sick on your injection day", whereas the forum and people on there got me through the two days a week I spent clutching a rubbish bin (even at the office) for dear life and feeling as though I had just eaten a cheese grater.

Through this forum, you inadvertently end up hearing about what treatments everyone is on – people in the States, Canada, the UK, Ireland, Australia and even The Netherlands. You come to make your own conclusions about the route of care and at which degree of disease aggression these routes change – no doctor can prepare you as much as watching and hearing the path of others going through it – at what point they were put on such and such and what it did for (and sometimes to) them. I learned that nearly everyone is put onto high dose steroids, many are additionally put onto heavy duty immunosuppressant's and that the really rough cases, like myself, tend to go onto Remicade (Infliximab) – the "miracle drug".

Remicade is a drug that is given by IV on a schedule of every month or six weeks and, along with a slew of other medical cocktail drugs, seems to be able to control the disease enough to eliminate steroids all together – sometimes even pushing the disease itself into remission. This is what I've gathered from the forum. However, it's not an approved drug for this disease (again. Yay for rare diseases, right?) because so few people get to the stage of needing this drug and no formal trials have yet been done on it. It is typically used for Chron's Disease and Rheumatoid Arthritis, with brilliant results for both.

I've got both a cousin and uncle back in Canada that suffer greatly from Chron's – both claim that Remicade almost immediately changed their lives. A friend of mine in Sweden also has Chron's – she told me that getting onto Remicade gave her back her life. The few people on the sarcoidosis forum that are on Remicade tout its greatness to no end – despite their multi-year struggles with their insurance companies to get on it in the first place. So, uplifted and sure that I had found a "cure" on the internet, I armed myself with all of the anecdotal evidence I could find (the best kind of evidence, surely) and burst into the office of my Rheumatologist asking about Remicade and how we can get this going.

Fortunately, this was already an option she was considering, but she explained to me how it worked in the UK – that it's not a drug that can just be prescribed for my condition, I had to "pass" (fail miserably) a number of tests before a funding application can even be made, at which point it could take months before the council makes a decision and the infusions could begin. This was in May of 2012. So, with Remicade in my view as a last (ultimate) resort, I followed her plan of high dose steroids and methotrexate at the maximum dose, cheese grater stomach and all. I was changed to something stronger than methotrexate, and after being hospitalized for yet another flare I was increased to the maximum possible dose of that as well. Hooray! I had completely failed two mainstream immunosuppressant therapies (passed! With flying colors! One of the most spectacular drug failures she had ever seen!) and we again discussed Remicade – with her promising to start a funding application for me immediately.

Unfortunately, as I'm sure you can see by now, things very rarely ever go in my favor.

Next came one of the worst flares of my life. The pain had been increasing steadily for about a week. My eyes burned in the light and my bones ached and seared with heat. My skin was red and hot to the touch above the parts of my cheeks, shins, hands, joints and bones as they burned. My legs felt as though they had been broken – that throbbing, aching pressure that radiates outward from a bone as it begins to heal after a break – in my face, my ribs, my wrists, my fingers and my shins, ankles and the tops of my feet. I could barely function. I felt I could barely breathe for the stabbing jolts rushing through my ribs as they expanded with each breath. The exhaustion had reached a new extreme – I was falling asleep like a narcoleptic pensioner all over the place. I couldn't think. I couldn't focus. I couldn't stop crying. I couldn't take it, and was brought into the hospital for another 13 day stay.

Crushingly, this put the miracle drug of Remicade off even further – as even the Professor of Rheumatology, the great, wise and undisputed leader of all Rheumatologists overseeing my care, came to my bed and told me that my disease had passed their remit and none of them had seen it like this before – it was time for me to be passed on to Dr. Sarc – a world renowned specialist in my disease at another London hospital, and they would continue to make me as comfortable as possible until I could see him.

I don't quite remember how I felt at that stage. There I was, alone again in a hospital bed with just my IV buddy and a room full of elderly, dying women – surrounded by six doctors, some students and two nurses all staring at the floor as their professor knelt beside my bed and told me that none of them could control this, that I was being passed on. I couldn't take the silence. I couldn't take the pity. And I couldn't cry in front of them.

So I looked him straight in the eye, winked and asked him if my 99 year old roommate on life support was going to out-live me and if so, should I tell my husband now to go ahead and start dating other people?

Thankfully, that even got a good, snorting laugh from one of my roommates that I had previously suspected had already passed and after my troupe of doctors left (chuckling and shaking their heads) I spent the next two days listening to her stories of growing up in Poland during the war and the years she spent living in the dug-out grave villages of Siberia with her children before being finally brought to the United Kingdom.

I decided right then that my life was really nothing to complain about and that really, I still had it pretty good.

I came out of that hospital stay with a heart full of hope and a brain full of mush – but who cares? I had an appointment with Dr. Sarc, the Brad Pitt of Rheumatology. I was more rabidly excited to see him than a Justin Bieber fan hiding in a hotel laundry cart. This was it. This is going to change everything.

A week passed and I hadn't heard anything. Yet another week passed. I saw my GP and broke down in her office in tears – she called his secretary right in front of me and urged her to squeeze me in faster. I hadn't even gotten the referral date yet. I wasn't even in their system. Didn't they realize that I was dying here? Didn't they realize that I've got a family and a life and a career? That everything in my life is hanging on a phone call, a letter, an email, an NHS text (I love those – but they really need to be more descriptive. Half the time I just do what the text says and rock up to an appointment with no idea of what test I'm about to be put through or person I'm about to see. I just line up at reception and hope to hell that at least *they* know what I'm there for).

Didn't they care?

He must care. I'm an interesting case, everyone has told me so. Med students love me. The Rheumatology Professor has written exam questions about me. I'm in a medical journal and two separate studies. He must know about me, right?

He didn't. I wasn't even in his system yet. I know. I called his poor receptionist, Joy, so much so that she must have considered a restraining order at one point or another. I finally broke down into choking sobs over the phone with her, begging for the earliest possible appointment and promising that I could get there on an hour's notice if need be – surely they have cancellations to be filled?

We have so much control in so many other aspects of our lives – what we do, who we see, when, how we feel, how we react to things. But this? When it comes to our health, when it comes to something like this – you're at the mercy of "the system". It's nearly unbearable to be able to do absolutely nothing about it. No letters I can write. No person I can talk to. No office I can call to chase up a result – just, wait. Hope and wait. Obsessively check the letterbox, refresh your emails… check if OCD is a side effect of any of your drugs…and wait.

In the end, Joy came through, and squeezed me in for

an appointment at the end of that very week. Amazing! I couldn't believe it. This was real. This was moving forward. This was *it*.

Oh, I had so many questions – so much to tell him. He would have answers, a plan! He would have seen other people like me, even people worse than me – that have come out the other side. I googled him and found his picture. I read his bio and his medical specialties and my heart skipped when it even listed Sarcoidosis – its very own listing and not just under "and other rare rheumatologic diseases". I told my family, my friends that I was going to see the Brad Pitt of Rheumatology, Dr. Sarc and I spent the rest of the week on Cloud Nine – excited, nervous but joyous. This was *it*!

My husband, on the other hand was trying to talk some sense into me (damn realist).

It might not work. He might not have all of the answers. He might not give you Remicade and even if he does, it might not work. Don't put all of your eggs in this one basket and other old clichés. He just didn't understand. He would though, and we arranged for him to come with me.

I think my well over the top excitement to see Dr. Sarc and all of the greatness and simplicity he would provide made the entire experience seem so much more surreal than it had to be. I remember arriving at the hospital with Paul – much earlier than I had to be and ready for the grandeur so suited and appropriate to a specialist such as this. We were directed to the basement and down halls of worn down, peeling yellow and green paint. We followed the red line sporadically painted throughout the maze of hallways and double doors meant to lead us to the Rheumatology department. The old fluorescent lights buzzed and flickered above us as we came to the end of the red line – a peeling, creaking and overloaded wooden desk where I gave my name and was directed by a hassled administrator to follow the blue painted line along the floor to the waiting area.

Obediently, we did so. No alarm bells going off yet, despite the scene we had walked into. Even when we turned the corner and saw two rows of old, oversized waiting chairs along each side of the corridor dotted with walkers, wheelchairs and the patrons more often clutching oxygen tanks than books or kindles. They all knew each other, as all elderly people seem to do, and chatted (wheezed) as the best of friends meeting for a coffee and a catch-up… until they saw me limp around the corner holding on to my husband for support. Every head turned, every conversation dulled. Again, I was clearly the youngest there by a good 30 years.

It was like a gazelle with a bit of a limp meandering smugly through a pack of toothless, arthritic lions.

You could hear what they were thinking from the looks on their faces.

"What's she doing here? Is she lost?"
"She *walked* here? Actually *walked*? What a hypochondriac"

and

"I've got a pacemaker older than this kid"

In the end I did what any self-respecting 31 year old Rheumatology patient would do – I ignored them, made a dramatic show of limping and wincing as I sat in my chair and pretended to play on my phone, despite having no reception or internet access in the cement hospital basement. I deserved to be here just as much as they did, I would see the great Dr. Sarc at last. I would get my answers, this whole thing was about to turn around. It was like waiting for an audience with the Wizard of Oz.

I started to sense something was up while watching Dr. Sarc's door. At first sighting when he came out to call in another patient it was like being star struck. I'd seen his picture online – he looked *exactly* like his picture online. My heart skipped a beat and I nearly jumped up with a felt tip pen asking him to sign my cleavage, despite him being A: Not a rockstar and B: an esteemed professional.

I managed to contain myself and remained in my oversized chair (it wouldn't be oversized to me for too much longer) and watched with rapt attention and increasing panic as the patients he called in stayed for no more than a minute or so before returning to the corridor to follow a particular colored line (Color blind people would be completely screwed down here. They must have to do a nightly grounds sweep for straggler color blind people as well as senile wanderers) to be replaced by the next patient being called in.

Nobody else was perturbed by this at all. I wondered why Dr. Sarc bothered to close the door to his office at all just to re-open it three minutes later to shuffle in the next poor, limping sap. I started actually timing his appointments on my phone's stop watch function. It was taking people more time to follow their colored lines down the hallway with their various walking and breathing aides than it was to see the doctor they came here to see.

I turned to Paul who had been too busy playing Angry Birds on his phone to notice anything was amiss. The panic in my eyes said everything – this was already not going to plan.

Dr. Sarc came out and called my name.

Oh God. I was no longer excited or nervous. I was scared. Scared that I was wasting his time, that I was really just a hypochondriac and that he would actually tell me so. Scared that he wouldn't even look at the list of symptoms and timeline of my condition that I had so carefully prepared last night. As I limped and lurched as quickly as I could through the corridor of well-aged judgment all coherent thoughts were left in my oversized chair down the hall. All of the questions I was ready to ask, all of the hope I had built up for this.

I hadn't even shaken this guy's hand yet and already it wasn't going well.

Nothing in life could have possibly prepared me for my initial three minute consultation with Dr. Sarc.

I was warmly welcomed into his small office and sat in a chair beside the desk he shared with his two assistants busily typing into their aged desktop computers, one not even glancing up as I entered the room. Dr. Sarc didn't shake my hand (he's a Rheumatologist, he knows that shaking hands is not only excruciating torture physically but also a grand way to ensure your patient's death by germs) but introduced himself and then more or less introduced me to myself as well out loud – giving me a brief synopsis of my condition and various hospital stays leading to his involvement – all the while speaking into a hand held recorder. He asked me two questions:

"You are a vegetarian?"

Yes.

"You have two year old fraternal twins conceived spontaneously?"

Umm… yes.

"Alright then. I agree that Remicade is going to be the next step for you, and I will put forth a funding application this week. Should take about six to eight weeks, you'll receive a notice to attend the infusion clinic at Charing Cross once it has been approved. Don't worry, we will take care of you."

Silence. Not, do you have any questions, is there anything you wanted to discuss, nothing. Silence. My cue to get up and leave, time for the next patient.

I thought of my list of carefully written out questions I had for him that was now crumpled and sweaty in my hand. My symptoms and how my condition had presented itself so suddenly, aggressively and severely compared to nearly everything I had read and how he must have treated and seen other people just like me – all of the things I was so desperate to know… nothing. I couldn't ignore the cue in that silence that I was out of time before I even had the chance to begin. I looked to Paul, tears already brimming in my eyes and he leaned forward, kissed me on the forehead, took my hand, politely thanked the doctor and his assistants for their time and led me back into the predatory hall to follow the colored line leading us to where we could make another appointment and where I could give more blood.

I cried in the car on the way home. Hard. Paul tried to comfort me, but there wasn't anything to say. I felt so helpless and defeated – all the hope I had pinned on this guy saving my life with a miracle had just been brutally extinguished. I meant nothing. I was a number. Another case file. A twin producing vegetarian to add to his research statistics.

That was all I was.

The very worst part was the realization that all of my other specialists and doctors were now just seeing me as part of a routine - none of them were any longer actively involved in my treatment as every single one of them, Rheumatologist, Pulmonologist, Neurologist, Virologist, Ophthalmologist – all of them were now putting their own ideas and decisions on hold and deferring to the great Dr. Sarc, who just dismissed me as though I didn't matter and wasn't worth more than three measly minutes of his time.

I was screwed.

This drug, Remicade, is not an approved drug for my disease. Anecdotally they know that it works. They've used it before, but my doctors can't prescribe it. It needs to go through the council, through a board, through a funding application. Probably through a subsequent appeal. None of which I have any control over, or can even contribute to. Dr. Sarc was on it, it was completely out of my hands.

So obediently I waited. And waited. The time frame I was given of six to eight weeks by Dr. Sarc passed. Then it doubled.

Did they forget about me? Had it gotten lost in the post? Should I call someone? Would I be an annoyance if I did? I again saw Dr. Sarc – an hour and a half each way on the tube for a three minute revolving door appointment in which I was simply told "I'll chase that up for you". Seriously. A phone call wouldn't have sufficed?

I waited more. A month more. Still nothing. I was getting desperate, I couldn't continue to live my life like this. My life of needing a nap after a particularly strenuous shower. My life of putting my kids in wellies just so I wouldn't have to wrestle their shoes onto their squirming feet. My life of inexplicably increasing girth on a diet that would starve a damn rabbit. Of mood swings and sweating in public like a prized pig in a sauna. My life of constant pain, fear and uncertainty.

People say a lot of stupid things when you get sick. It's hard to fault them for it, I've said stupid things to sick people too – we all do. Things like "it could be worse" or "that's not *so* bad". It was recently pointed out to me that true empathy rarely begins with 'at least'. Yes, I am fully aware that being mauled by an AIDS carrying, rabid mountain lion is 'worse', but that hardly means that being diagnosed with my disease is great. Being diagnosed with a rare condition that nobody has really ever heard of tends to produce some doozies – like my favorite "at least it's not cancer". What they don't realize when they say it is that you often wish it was. At least that is something known, something that you can count on. You know what the treatment will be, you know what the outcome might be… you know. With this so much is unknown, unstudied, unfunded. You also hear a lot of "but you don't look sick" or "you look great" – which is a compliment at any rate, but stings beneath the reality of how you are feeling. Much worse when even your doctors don't know what to do with you. You are moved from specialist to specialist or, in my experience, they are brought to you in hospital – a constant stream of being studied and initial reactions of "my med students would *love* to see this". Funny, yes. Comforting, not so much. I was in limbo – my various doctors all waiting on the advice of Dr. Sarc, with Dr. Sarc waiting on the funding application. What could possibly be said other than "I'm sorry, we will just have to wait." How stabbing those few words have become.

And so I waited.

Then something happened that nobody could ignore – I had a stroke at the age of 32. You just can't explain that away, and my preferred coping mechanism of blind denial took a major hit.

Even though having a stroke certainly *helped*, it's not a strategy I would outright recommend. I left the hospital a week later with the promises of the doctors there to chase up my funding application and that they would urge Dr. Sarc themselves to push the funding application. It was my own doctor that, watching me finally succumb to defeat in her faded, worn office chair, had a more direct approach.

Together we found online that Dr. Sarc also worked privately at a clinic downtown, perhaps I could indeed push this along. Private doctor? As well as working in the NHS? Could a person do that? Being from Western Canada this concept blew my mind. Wait, you could get *Remicade* privately? Exactly how much was this going to cost? I inundated my GP with questions about how this worked but she didn't know – she gave me the website of Dr. Sarc's private clinic in Central London and asked me to keep her updated – I left so distracted with this new realm of possibilities that I sat in her washroom for 20 minutes before remembering that my husband, children and dog were waiting for me out in the car.

I got home and researched frantically, attempting to determine how much this drug would be privately, as well as how I would possibly pay for it. I was told figures ranging from £15,000 a month, £8,000, £4,000... I felt like a Price is Right contestant where all of the other contestants secretly work for the same drug company and I'm actually in an unknown negotiation in which the more people I ask the cheaper it seemed to get. Everybody had a different answer, and I was considering asking the hospital phlebotomist for her opinion in the hope that she knows someone that knows someone that hands it out the back of an NHS pharmacy for the simple exchange of one of my non-vital organs and a fiver. I had been forced into sobriety by my medication anyway – what did I really need both kidneys for?

I wanted this, badly, but was having mixed feelings about the concept of private care. Being from Canada we take great pride in our healthcare system in that the care is good and you are seen regardless of social status or financial wealth. I firmly believe in this, that my financial position makes no assertion as to my value as a human being when it comes to quality of healthcare and sustaining my life, nor does it to anyone else. Everyone deserves to be cared for, and we shouldn't be able to jump the queue at the cost of someone else just because I could afford to do so.

But I couldn't continue to live like this. Perhaps I would just call his private secretary and feel it out.

What followed was surely the most bizarre and convoluted enquiry this poor woman has ever received.

"Hi, um… is this Dr. Sarc's office?"

"Yes, how can I help you?"

"His (whispers) *private* office?" (in my mind it was a bit of a dirty word)

"… Yes. Can I help?"

"I have Sarcoidosis, and I see Dr. Sarc on the NHS, we are waiting for drug funding but I wanted to find out about having this drug done privately, do you do Remicade at the clinic?"

"We do, yes. Have you got insurance?"

"Oh, I can get insurance for this?"

"Um, probably not at this stage, no."

"Ah yes. I'm more uninsurable than a narcoleptic skydiver now"

"… um … well, you can pay out of pocket but it tends to be extremely expensive so very few people choose to go that route, Remicade at the clinic averages about £2000 per month. "

"That's it?! Sign me up! When can I come in?!!!"

"You need to have a consultation with Dr. Sarc first, which is an additional £220 for half an hour."

"I get a whole half hour?! That's amazing! How do I book?"

She seemed rather surprised at my reaction, and explained to me that she could book me in for that evening at 8:00pm if I'd like, she would send over for my electronic notes and I was to bring anything I had with me as he may not remember me without my details. I was elated, but suddenly nervous again.

"Can I ask one more thing?"

"Of course. How can I help?"

"Is he going to be mad at me?"

I swear I could hear crickets in the background. In my mind I was jumping the queue. I was being unfair, I was cheating his other patients. Private care was not for me, someone who was already getting adequate care on the NHS and should be happy with what I was given. Private care was for wealthy Russian entrepreneurs and their gorgeous wives, for celebrities and people that could use the NHS but didn't want the hassle of paparazzi following them to give blood samples. Who was I to demand his attention? Who was I to declare my condition worse than another's, myself more deserving? What would he think of me when he recognized me as an NHS patient – that I was a demanding hypochondriac? A desperate lunatic? A spoiled brat hypocrite contributing to the failure of the public system? Would he file a restraining order? Even worse – I'm used to everything being done in three minutes with Dr. Sarc, how could I even fill an entire half hour? What if we just sat there and stared at each other in silence? How do you even make small talk with a doctor?

I focused my thoughts then on how I was going to pay for this treatment – I was seeing him in six hours and I needed a plan. I called my husband to consult – to him as well it wasn't a question of 'if' but 'how' – this was important and we needed to do it. Debt? Sell the car? Send my husband, a stay at home dad, back to work? Prostitution (his)? Take in another roommate? Let a group of Gypsies move into the back garden? Incidentally it wouldn't be the first time we'd found a group of Gypsies living in our back garden.

I needed to talk to my boss, who was about to meet me at an outrageously expensive block of flats outside of the London Eye – he wanted me to move my family downtown so I would be closer to the office and thus this would somehow improve my illness. He would pay for the difference in price – so was carting me from property to property to find a suitable flat between the price range of very expensive and stupidly expensive when I asked if perhaps instead of paying for a flat that

I'd not really like he could pay to keep me alive instead. He very generously offered to pay for both but I didn't want to move. I don't understand how Americans can function like this – to have my health and my very existence now linked to my employment. It was bad enough that should I lose my job I would be deported but now if I lost my job I would be deported and my medical treatment withdrawn. I'd not stopped working at all throughout my ordeal with Sarc, but maintaining my high achieving workaholism had now literally become a matter of life and death.

The rest of my day descended into an obsession of seeing Dr. Sarc that evening. I even arranged for my boss to come with me as I couldn't handle this level of stress and anticipation on my own. I didn't know what I was going to say – I so badly feared that Dr. Sarc would be disappointed in me for having 'gone private'. I felt as though I was counting down the hours until my life might suddenly change. I imagined the sky suddenly clearing as I opened the clinic doors to burst outside in song. Doves flying from the open clinic windows as I musically bounded down the front steps and into the street, a well-choreographed troupe of dancing strangers joining me in celebration of sudden freedom and health. This could be it, I could be myself again by just eight o'clock tonight. I imagined Dr. Sarc in his private practice as a closeted faith healer in flowing white robes holding a telethon fundraiser for those in need of a miracle. I practically skipped to his office, oblivious to my surroundings and was nearly mowed down by a London double decker bus as I pranced about.

Maybe I ought to settle down a bit.

There could be a down side to this as well. What if it didn't work? What if he doesn't give me the miracle drug? Could I continue to live the way I am? What if my body, my life, doesn't get any better than this? What if it gets worse? My husband hates the 'what if's' with a passion, and when I descend into the pit of endless 'what if's' he asks me ridiculous things like: "What if aliens invaded in the 70's and we were never born?"

Wait, what?

"Exactly."

He uses this to prove that 'what if's' are pointless and something that shouldn't be worried about. I think it just proves that he's an ass. He's right, however, as there isn't much point in dwelling on what if's. No amount of 'what if's' could have prepared me for that appointment with Dr. Sarc – which kicked off my great 'chemo race' and a whole other chapter of wild adventures.

And whilst seeing him privately he was actually quite pleasant and nice. And he doesn't hate me for singlehandedly undermining the entirety of the National Health Service.

Probably.

Empowerment is overrated

Internet forums can be a confusing place to gather information and support, particularly as they now rarely stick within the confines of national borders. As is common with rare disease a single forum will stand out with members contributing from across the globe with their experience and stories. I've met a few of these forum members in person now – in the Netherlands and within the UK – though the site seems to be dominated by Americans with their own unique perspective on healthcare, which is often confusing and always entertaining.

In one instance a British member had expressed that she was frustrated with her consultant, who she found to be abrasive, dismissive and extremely rushed. She didn't feel that she could talk through her concerns with him and was feeling frustrated, asking other forum members for advice in dealing with him. An American responded, explaining that she won't keep a doctor if she doesn't leave their office feeling empowered and enthusiastic about her treatment. She suggested that this person talk to her consultant again, saying that she expected him to make her feel empowered and appreciated or she would find another doctor. After all, the doctor was essentially working for *her* and she expected a certain standard of service along with it.

I messaged the poster to find that the consultant she was referring to actually was my own Dr. Sarc, and we howled in laughter just imagining sitting him down for a conversation about the expectation for him to make us feel more empowered when really, we had been passed to him for the purpose of just keeping us alive at this point. I wouldn't dream of giving Dr. Sarc a 'talking to' – other than to thank him profusely for all that he has done for me so far. And neither could she.

Even his junior doctors seem terrified of Dr. Sarc who is, admittedly, so busy and efficient that he has not one but two secretaries with him at all times. His Registrar, Dr. Navo was once chatting with me up on the ward whilst putting an IV line into my arm. He jiggled it around a bit and said "I think it's in." Being an unrelenting wise-ass I cracked a joke about how it is never comforting to hear "I think" when someone is talking about your veins and sharp objects. Dr. Navo sat back and burst into laughter, apologizing and confiding that Dr. Sarc *hates* hearing "I think" and will challenge it relentlessly and publicly. "You think? You *think*?!" until you are nearly in tears and shouting back "No! I know! I *know*!"

He may not have the greatest bedside manner or patient soothing skills but with his ability to control what ails us I'll stick with the specialist with the manner of an aloof badger, thanks. Empowerment is highly overrated.

The Guy From The Apprentice Hates Me

As I continued to struggle with the residual weight gain effects of my steroid treatments, Dr. Sarc suggested referring me to a specialist dietician at another private hospital in which he worked, in St. John's Wood of

London. Desperate to try anything to combat my steroid weight and having not yet heard back from the NHS Dietician referral team for over a year I struggled a lot less with this decision to go private. So off I went to meet with this dietician who, like Dr. Sarc when going privately – could suddenly fit me in that very evening.

The dietician is a wonderful woman, kind yet firm and she put me onto what I affectionately call the Prisoner of War diet. It has restricted pretty much everything imaginable but it works so I'm hardly about to complain. She explained to me that it was not my fault, I wasn't eating bad foods or over eating. I couldn't understand why my friends could gorge on fast food and fizzy drinks yet not gain a pound while I would gain six just *thinking* about a cupcake. "It's the steroids" she said, "not you." And she was right – the steroid infusions I was being given would easily put on 10 pounds in a week without any other change. I was active and walked often, ate well and took care of myself in a healthy manner but again, I was looking like Jabba the Hut in Drag regardless. Now *there* is a doctor that leaves you feeling empowered.

I arrived to see her at a clean white hospital just outside the underground station – my first hint of what I was about to be in for came from asking the concierge standing at the door for direction, at which point he gestured for someone to snap to my side and personally walk me to my appointment. Which was great, because this place was far too posh for signage. We came to pass even more reception desks, each with crisply suited staff smiling a greeting and ensuring that I didn't require anything at all.

We traipsed up the stairs and to the waiting room full of aesthetically placed black armchairs around pristine glass coffee tables boasting the latest copy of the Times and Forbes. Patients waiting were offered coffees and teas and, rather than having to take a number and wait your turn for a blood test a Phlebotomist came out to personally invite you to please come with them to have your blood taken, and have you been offered a coffee?

Other patients watched the news being played on the large screen television mounted on the wall and still others sat back to read the many international newspapers available. Consultants and doctors came out of their respective offices to collect their patients themselves, greeting them all with handshakes and warm smiles like old friends. This was certainly… different.

I've so far only encountered one celebrity there, however, and he hates me. The star of the Apprentice and all around well-heeled entrepreneur, hates me. I don't know why, I'm not even one to stare. Having lived in China as a tall white blonde woman I get what it's like to be stared at and hounded (I once had a woman run up behind me at Tiananmen Square and cut off a piece of my hair as a souvenir) and I'd not like to make anyone else, famous or not, feel so uncomfortable. But that man just stares you down for daring to glance in his direction. I've seen him there on three separate occasions and he just glares at me, as though daring me to come up and ask him for business advice or something. I'm not interested, I'm there for my own issues thanks – but that man's hatred of me has turned him into my own private hospital nemesis.

And everyone needs one of those. If you don't already have one I would highly recommend it.

I have since come to greatly appreciate the collaborative system of public and private healthcare in the United Kingdom – a wonderful and robust public system with an affordable and efficient private side-step should a patient wish to pursue care at a quicker and more personalized pace. The NHS is truly a beautiful thing that deserves to be protected and appreciated. From an outsider's perspective as a patient this has been a frightening journey with the best care I could have ever anticipated.

So thank your doctors, your consultants and the junior doctors that are doing what they can in a difficult system. Appreciate the nurses that treat you with kindness and compassion despite being run off their feet and buried in so much paperwork that they can barely do the job they got into in the first place. Be nice to the people that make the whole thing run – the receptionists and support staff, the cleaning staff and the people that come by just to offer you some hot tea and a biscuit – because the system here is unique and grand in so many ways.

I'd not want to be ridiculously diseased anywhere else.

Chapter Seven: You've Just Got to Laugh

There's very little that can happen during my day at work that cannot be remedied by an amusing ride home on public transport.

Being a wee bit paranoid about the drastic and consistent suppression of my immune system, particularly enhanced by my current chemotherapy, I started wearing a SARS mask – on the tube.

At first I tried finding some decent quality facial masks that looked somewhat socially acceptable or at least reasonably inconspicuous online, but didn't actually find very much. Having lived in China I knew that these things existed – cloth, washable facial masks that covered your mouth and nose by hooking around your ears but alas, not many to be found in the United Kingdom online. I asked my doctor about them and she, agreeing that this was probably a good idea, directed me to my local pharmacy – who sold me a box of 24 masks for a mere couple of pounds. They were paper surgical masks – possibly only slightly less alarming in than wearing a fully functioning gas mask on public transportation.

My first trip wearing one I was very nervous. Would everyone stare? Of course they would – I would. It was winter, could I possibly cover it a bit with my bulky yet fashionable scarf? Not all the way, though I tried many different stylings in the mirror before leaving the house.

191

I didn't need it for the walk *to* the tube, just once I was actually on the tube – so I kept it tucked away in my pocket until then, crowding onto the train with the rest of the rush hour commuters with heads buried in books and newspapers.

Well, whipping out and putting on a surgical mask on a packed train is certainly one way to get a quick seat.

Plenty of room too, as absolutely nobody would sit beside or across from me. On a packed tube during rush hour I had my own little oasis of personal space – why hadn't I thought of doing this *years* ago? After a few stops the stares started to become unnerving – as more people got on, couldn't believe their luck at finding an empty seat and then recoiled back to the sardine pit of the area between the train doors. People looked, pretending not to stare – averting their eyes to the breasts of the person next to them if I made eye contact. Others stared openly, some pointed. I felt defiant – clearly I was not wearing this as a fashion statement (or was I?), clearly there was something wrong with me and clearly it was communicable (it wasn't, but it is much more fun to let people believe that it is).

Upon arriving at my office I took out the mask and with a black felt tip pen wrote:

'It's not for my protection, it's for yours.'

Take that staring London commuters.

That went over reasonably well, some laughed, some

scoffed and others switched trains at the next available station. I was at least having a bit of defiant fun with it, and was sat there on the busy tube home with my SARS mask and scarf, head in a book when my ride home suddenly became much more interesting.

A woman and her husband boarded the busy train, upset that she had to stand in the corridor of the train as all of the seats were full. Quite a number of people were already standing quietly and patiently, the type of thing common on British public transport. This woman would *not* stop letting her distaste be known. She made loud, pointed remarks to her husband about everything and everyone – the 'perfectly well looking man sleeping in the priority seat'. The man that gave up his seat to an elderly woman instead of her, even though she had *clearly* been on the train for much longer. Shooting daggers, furious at a young mother for having dared to bring her pushchair on the train during peak hours. She tsk'd about this and tsk'd about that – staring at seated passengers as though challenging them for their precious seat. I, sat in my SARS mask, was having a great time watching the inadvertent show this woman was putting on – and then things got even *better*.

The train pulled into White City – a large outdoor station on the Central Line and, just before the doors closed, a raving crazy woman jumped on board. She was there to spread the word of the Lord Jesus whether we were willing participants or not, knowing full well that she had a good three full minutes before we arrived at the next station and our first opportunity to make a run for it off the train. She shouted the righteousness of the Almighty God and warned us of the fiery hell that awaited the non-believers. People backed up to the doors, as far as they could go – even some gave up their coveted seats – the scoffing woman not even moving forward to secure that which she had pined for so badly. The crazed woman sat next to me and hurled verses and prayers to passengers down the train – "You with the brown coat! Jesus loves you and died for your sins!" and "You with the glasses! He loves you and made you in his image! Repent or burn in the eternal fires!"

See, this was going rather well for me as the SARS mask nicely covered first my shock and then my grinning laughter at the whole scene. Oddly enough I seemed to be the only one smiling and having a good time with this, trembling with awkward giggles poorly disguised as coughs. This drew the attention of the Bible clutching woman – who told me that Jesus heals all if only I believed as I nodded along enthusiastically. This continued for six more stops, with people jumping off the train at their next opportunity and people jumping on only to realize their mistake once the doors had already firmly closed.

The crazed woman prepared to disembark at the next stop and just before the doors opened she shouted to us all "Bless you! Jesus loves you and I love you and please repent your sins, opening your arms to the almighty!" In response to the shocked, silent looks throughout the captive crowd I threw my arms up in the air and shouted "Amen!" after her and to the gawking passengers – a grand finale to the night's commuting entertainment. I looked down at the rest of the train, lowered my mask and declared "Why not? It's not like we get TV down here!", releasing the pent up tension and relaxing the crowd as they burst into giggles and smiles of camaraderie at what we had just witnessed and endured.

Madame Bitchypants nearly scoffed herself to death.

Facebook

Although somewhat complimentary, I never know how to take it when hospital ward staff say "Oh hey, it's you! Welcome back!"

Medication everywhere yet not a vegetable in sight

When it comes to food I will never understand how it is that hospitals are about the most unhealthy places with a captive audience. This has become somewhat of a soapbox issue for me since becoming ill, when in desperation I looked to food as a natural form of healing. Perhaps it couldn't cure me, but surely it could help. It was within this change of heart that I came across Lisa and her blog www.100daysofrealfood.com in which Lisa presents simple yet profoundly logical ideas about how what we eat has changed and that really, if your great-grandparents wouldn't recognize it as food you shouldn't be eating it. Since reading this blog we as a family have cut back dramatically on our processed food – our home is filled with vegetables and fruits, whole grains and the proper ingredients to make food – gone are our freezer drawers stocked with instant meals, frozen pizzas and magnum ice creams (okay I lied. The Magnums are still in there sometimes). We *like* this new way of eating – we feel better, have more energy and our kids aren't sugar filled demons hell-bent on world domination and despair. This way of eating certainly hasn't cured me, far from it, but we all feel better for it and wouldn't dream of going back to how we had eaten before.

If given the choice.

Now, when you are in the hospital and your husband is sneaking you in fruit and vegetables this might be an indication that the health system needs a bit of work.

I vaguely remember hospital food back in Western Canada as being a set meal of chicken, fish or vegetarian with the cursory Jell-O cup afterward. In China the hospital food was much better – hot rice with vegetables and then some kind of meat or tofu. Probably. I wasn't very good at identifying it back then and was really much more bothered by the state of the washrooms and hallways in the hospital there than I was the food. The hospital food in the United Kingdom, however, surprised me as I was presented with a menu.

A menu.

A colorfully presented five page menu of choices for each meal, plus snacks. There wasn't just a vegetarian option, there were vegetarian options! Plural! Now, for any vegetarian this is a rather overwhelming presentation – I then had the further option of western vegetarian, halal vegetarian, Indian vegetarian and even Caribbean vegetarian. It was too overwhelming for me – as a western vegetarian I am much more accustomed to my restaurant options being limited to the one vegetarian item or a salad, hold the chicken. And so began my despairing love affair with the NHS's macaroni and cheese that was suspiciously lacking in macaroni – with a side of peas.

Menu or not though, this was still hospital food.

I soon grew tired of my macaroni suspiciously lacking in macaroni – and after Day 5 of the same meal for lunch and dinner alike I started to venture toward other vegetarian meal choices – I really had nothing better to look forward to during my stay and figured that at least trying every vegetarian curry item on the menu would keep the overenthusiastic enema nurse away from me. Hopefully.

I've never been a big fan of spicy food, though having lived in China for a number of years in my youth taught me a thing or two about handling spicy food with grace. Having arrived in China without a word of Chinese to my brain I quickly armed myself with the most necessary of words and phrases such as 'help!' and 'tofu' by asking a Chinese colleague. Instead of a standard 'help' he taught me the equivalent of 'save my life!' which was a lot of fun in grocery stores as I unknowingly shouted 'save my life where are the green beans?!' at passers-by that didn't actually work there. In an equally dramatic style this colleague was not content to simply give me basic words like 'help' and 'tofu' – I had to ask for a *kind* of tofu. He didn't ask me what kind I might like, just told me that tofu was 'mapo dofu' - I could remember that, surely. Turns out it meant 'fire tofu' or, more aptly, 'burn your face off tofu' but, being the only food related word I knew at the time how to say and having completely failed at charade-vegetable restaurant orders I continued to order mapo dofu at the same restaurant for every single meal for an entire week, tears running down my red face, nose running and yelping in starved misery. The restaurant staff thought I was insane (or that all foreigners were insane) as I would come in twice a day, every day, place my order and burst into tears. I didn't think anything could be worse than Chinese fire tofu. The NHS proved me wrong.

See, a green bean masala *sounds* innocent enough. Who doesn't like green beans? Or masala? Win win! I figured it sounded the most familiar and was eager to give it a try. It came in some kind of microwaved ready meal package with a plastic covering, just a rectangular black bowl of green beans hiding in a dark brown sauce – the odd chick pea here and there. I had declined the rice, leaving just the masala and an orange for lunch on my depressing little plastic tray. My roommates tucked in to their scrumptiously grease ridden fish and chips, mashed potatoes and sausages, chips and pot pies. I looked over at them, smug with my healthy Indian vegetarian selection as I peeled back the melting plastic and dug in my spoon for a heaping mouthful of sweet, creamy masala...

That was *not* masala. That was surely ground up

liquefied chili peppers prepared in the fires of hell. My mouth was aflame – I couldn't feel my lips. My tongue burned as I sputtered and grabbed for the water pitcher by my bed, chugging it down like a deranged madwoman straight from the spout, splashing it down my front. I didn't care, I just wanted the burning to stop. This made the burning so, so much worse. So much worse. The only other thing I had to coat my mouth and take away this pain was the orange – which I grabbed and started to rip apart with my fingernails in frantic desperation. My roommates had all stopped eating and were staring at the spectacle that was me, my hyperventilating having risen to the pitch of a high, staccato dolphin-like whine. I couldn't even speak, my mouth was on fire. I put the first chunk of orange into my mouth – that was even worse! The acid from the orange made it somehow so much worse. I had reached a whole new level of searing, burning pain and I looked around ready to leap out of bed to shamelessly steal bread or anything that could quell the burning should any of my elderly roomies have some in sight but I was tied to the bed by machines… I could go nowhere. I couldn't even call for a nurse!

I had reached an entirely new level of frantic desperation as, having absolutely no other solution come to mind, the nurse finally walked in to find me in bed on all fours leaning forward and licking my hospital bed sheet like a dog in an attempt to scrape the remaining hellfire masala off my tongue in front of my laughing 80 year old ward-mates.

In a gown with no back, none the less.

I have since developed a whole new appreciation for NHS macaroni and cheese suspiciously lacking in macaroni – and went back to my routine of ordering this for both lunch and dinner – with my husband bringing in the odd contraband container of fresh cut pineapple or tofu with fresh veggies. I even at times shared my preciously healthful loot with other patients in the next beds – like cellmates in a Colombian prison having just had family members slip fresh burritos through the window, quickly stuffing our faces with kiwi and steamed cauliflower with hummus - the paper curtains pulled around us in secrecy.

I will never fully understand the food in hospitals. I grasp that processed food is cheap and that this is a critical cost saving measure, yet surely the long term goal of educating people on healthful eating as well as helping their healing along while in hospital with good food gets them out faster, no? If they eat well in hospital and are then discharged to run straight into the nearest fast food joint that can't be helped, but an apple here and there might get them out of hospital quicker and at the very least save a bit for the NHS on constipation meds.

During one of my week long stays in hospital a policy change took place as a cost saving measure – patients were given hot breakfasts and lunches with a cold dinner – like a boxed sandwich dinner. We were told about it being implemented the next day, as patients, and that this hospital trust was going to be doing it as a trial. No big deal, it's just food. I doubt anyone rebelled too violently at the news and we all looked forward to seeing what the next day's dinner would bring. You don't get a whole lot of excitement as an in-patient outside of the psych ward, so we were genuinely looking forward to the excitement.

To my surprise, as a vegetarian I was given an egg and cheese sandwich on white bread, in a box, with a bag of lays potato chips and a can of diet coke.

By dinner time at 5:30 the very next day the ward door was buzzing non-stop with a constant stream of delivery drivers from Dominoes, Pizza Hut, curry houses, Chinese takeaways and even a fish and chip shop. My own husband brought two pizzas from Papa John's, one for me and one for the nursing station – the nurses only got a few slices out of the box before it was descended upon in a hostile takeover from a group of elderly men across the hall – one being 'crazy Willy in Wellies' who really, you don't argue with as he'd spent two hours earlier that day yelling obscenities at his own boots for 'looking at him funny'.

The patients were laughing (most of us – well, those that hadn't yet had their senses of humor surgically removed) as the entire ward looked like it was recovering from a wild college party – we'd never been so well fed. Pizza boxes towered in the spaces beside rubbish bins already overstuffed with takeaway boxes. Patients wandered around in slippers and robes pushing along their IV poles to mingle and check out what the other rooms had ordered for takeout. The few that didn't order anything either pouted on their beds with their sandwiches and crisps or got up and offered to pitch in for the now many varieties of pizza being passed around. That's one way to get people's spirits up in an 'infectious disease' ward! We laughed, we gathered around the beds of those that were trapped there. Someone's husband brought M&S chocolates and the party really got started – though the nurses intervened when a couple of women attempted to order out for wine. We swapped stories of horrid hospital food, the story of me licking my bed-sheet earlier in the week had apparently made it all the way down the hall and into other rooms. We laughed about other patients and compared surgical scars. It was quite a sight, this party of elderly seniors and me, a good 40 years their junior and having the time of my life. The evening med nurse arrived with her ancient wooden cart of medicinal goodies which, once she finally located each of us in turn, we compared with the gusto of exotic bar cocktails – still laughing and threatening to swap meds with each other to see what would happen.

From what I remember the hospital brought back hot dinners to our ward the very next day.

In other trips to the hospital, even just for appointments and day ward visits (my life is clearly very exciting) this theme has continued. Restaurants serve chips and vegetables smothered in cheese sauce. Nothing whole wheat and everything in a heavy cream. Royal Free Hospital does a brilliant vegetable stir fry that I suspect brings in diners that aren't even near the hospital for lunch as it is so good and so cheap – but otherwise as a vegetarian the options are limited to blocks of cheese or greasy fridge samosas from the bookstore at the entrance, brownies and pizza pockets from the coffee shop or, in one London hospital, Burger King. Has a hospital really become a place in which healthful food is actually obsolete? Is the promotion of long term dietary health as preventative medicine really not best situated in a hospital? I don't get it, and I never will.

But despite my veggie soapbox, the NHS has kind of hooked me on their macaroni and cheese suspiciously lacking in macaroni. It may not be the healthiest thing on the menu, but it's actually not that bad. The last time I was brought into A&E for a flare one of the first things I asked a nurse was whether or not upon being admitted I'd be too late to order dinner.

I'll have the macaroni please.

The Sidewalk Starfish

Clearly we have to move.

I've been feeling pretty good lately so, with a rare spring in my step I've been walking home from the tube each day after work rather than taking the bus or having my husband pick me up – as I can feel my body getting stronger. I've got more energy, I have the urge to stretch neglected muscles and can feel the fullness of fresh air in my lungs. I was walking home thinking about how fantastic I felt and how great I was (oh admit it, you've done it too), walking like a normal person at a normal pace, finally holding my bag as though it was more out of fashion than gripped necessity and then-

Wham!

Man down! Woman down! Tripping on *nothing* I was up, not a single body part touching the ground – I was flying, propelling forward in an instinctive roll that turned into more of a maniacal cartwheel of doom that launched my bag out into the street. I came to the ground hard like a wobbly sack of jelly, skidding along the sidewalk on my knees having done a complete forward flip. I came to a halt, face-down on the pavement and turned my head in horror to watch as my laptop, iPad, iPhone and wallet tore out of my bag and further into the street.

I made to push myself up to scurry into the street to retrieve my things, my precious i-things, but my legs… they wouldn't work. I couldn't move them at all past getting up to sit back on my knees. (my poor, bleeding knees) The impact had shocked my joints and bones, already flaring from sarc – and I couldn't make them work. I couldn't stand. I couldn't even crawl. I was terrified and hurt and humiliated. I had literally fallen and couldn't get up. Like some sort of diseased turtle.

What to do? Tough it out? Laugh it off as a crowd of strangers rushed to the aid of the fat lady splayed face down and sobbing on the sidewalk surrounded by Apple devices? Oh no. No no no no no.

I started to cry.

Not just a little bit, a lot. Tears pouring down my face.

That high pitched, only dogs and dolphins can understand what you are saying type of cry. More of a hysterical wail. My shoulders heaved with wracking sobs. I could almost see my house but couldn't get there – I couldn't get off my knees. I was completely and utterly defeated, Sarc had gotten me.

A very lovely young Indian couple collected my things and offered to call me an ambulance. I politely declined (I think. I intended to decline, certainly, but God knows what actually came out of my high pitched opera of despair and humiliation in the middle of my street) and I waved them off. They left, reluctantly, as did everyone else once they were certain that I had all of my things, knew where I lived and my firm assurances that I would be fine, I was just resting.

I eventually made it to my feet like some sort of belligerent penguin insistent on erecting myself independently, complete with racking sobs and shocked gasps from the remaining small crowd of eight or so elderly neighbors as the amount of blood pooled beneath me became visible. (blood thinners have proven to be highly entertaining). I again assured the crowd that I was fine, I 'always bleed like that' and that I was sure it would wash off the sidewalk during the next rain.

My bags were handed back to me, I put on my brave face and politely thanked everyone for their help but assured them once again that I was alright, I was nearly home anyway. I pushed all of the pain down and shuffled, zombie-like, toward my house- met halfway

205

by my jerk cat yowling gleefully at my ordeal and distress before running ahead to leap through an open kitchen window – presumably to have a good laugh about me with the dog before I got in (furry ingrates). My husband opened the door to find me standing at the door crying, bleeding and barely holding it together.

I burst into the house and into his arms wailing "I fell dowwwwwwwnnnn!!!!" He also offered to call me an ambulance – I felt it was best not to look down at my knees as the word 'ambulance' had been tossed around a bit too frequently to be ignored.

My husband sat me down onto the stairs like a child, taking my bag and coat, carefully pulling off my jeans and fetching a cold cloth and some peroxide. Being gently cleaned up and cared for so sweetly had a serene calming effect, reducing my sobs to mere hiccups of distress. I told him everything. From the dramatic cartwheel to the flying i-paraphanelia and the kindness of the crowd that wouldn't leave me alone to collect the shattered remnants of my pride.

He agreed with me that it would probably be best to move, though we did really love the area. Perhaps a blessing that the neighbors are quite old and most will have forgotten the incident completely on their way home anyway due to general senility.

The worst part of it all was that I ripped to shreds the only pair of jeans that still fit me. Well, that and that it didn't actually rain for a good week, so my bloodstains became a regular neighborhood attraction for a little while.

Humiliating.

The Support Group

I am finding it a common basic need to seek out and associate with like-people in even the most basic situations, not least of which upon becoming 'diseased'. The problem with a rare condition, however, is that these people also tend to be fairly spread out, resorting to coming together online in various forms of support and camaraderie. After nearly a year of going it on my own I searched for and found an online forum dedicated to those with my condition – Sarcoidosis. This site is hosted by Inspire, an online forum community for a wide variety of medical conditions in which people may be pulled together.

I'm not sure why 'Inspire' was the best description for such a forum, as I'm not sure it is meant to be inspiring. It is simply a forum for people that have something in common – I'm sure that 'miserable diseased gits' was on the table at some point but the powers that be went with something more ambiguous and uplifting (misleading), hence 'Inspire'. Regardless, it has become a place with active members from all over the globe discussing our shared condition and helping each other to effectively cope. It is also a place for some delightful dramatics – which is really what keeps me coming back week after week.

Through the forum I learned of an *actual* support group held regularly in London – how exciting! An opportunity to really meet other people with my condition, to talk it through and learn from their experience! Real people! I had never met anyone else with Sarc in person and felt that this was important to me, though I couldn't put my finger on why. It didn't matter, I was ready – and I signed up to attend.

My very first (and last!) Sarcoidosis support group meeting nearly broke out into a fistfight. Seriously. I know that I attract the crazy like stink to a monkey but this one surprised even me.

I had never before been to a support group meeting of any kind. I once, upon having just recently arrived in London, gave meetup.com a try in an attempt to find like-minded friends but that was an unmitigated disaster. The only group I felt I could identify with was the vegetarian group – out of a gathered friendless crowd of roughly 80 met outside a park I was quite possibly the only one there without dreadlocks and a guitar screaming about meat being murder or something about vegetable harmony.

This was different, though. I wasn't looking for friends, I was looking for support and validation from like-minded people also living with this condition. I now knew about the group, meeting once a month, but due to a combination of being too ill, too callous and, if I'm honest, too scared, I never went. Every month I found an excuse not to go. Had to work late, was too tired, too sore, it was too far...

So on a Thursday night I looked myself in the mirror at work and decided to go. I needed this. I had been feeling so good lately from my new treatments that I had more than enough energy and at the prompting of my husband (saying that if, as a worst case scenario, I don't personally get anything out of it at the very least I'll probably get a good story out of it) off I went. I got lost on the way there (of course I did) and was the last to arrive to a meeting already underway.

This was the most eclectic group of people I had ever envisioned. About twelve people, both men and women and, I was saddened to see, all thinner than I was. And with more hair.

Damn.

There was this one guy (there always is) and I should have known that something was up with him the moment I walked in and sat down - I was silent and sat there for about five minutes or so before he would even stop talking long enough for me to introduce myself. This guy was just off the wall. Had I really just signed myself up for two hours of listening to one person moan about how horrid his life and marriage was?

To make it even worse, the hospital had a signal blocker, rendering it impossible to discreetly play on Facebook with my phone under the table. So I scrolled through my pictures. Played a game for a bit. Checked my already downloaded emails. Contemplated pretending to have Tourette's, making a scene and bolting for the door.

I looked around the table - it wasn't just me. Two others had their phones under the table and the rest had that glossy eyed "checked out" look going on.

He was still talking. Something about him being a ninja now. And how his wife hates him. Oh man, it was awkward. Oh wow, it somehow got worse. He was like a train-wreck in slow motion. He was talking about his mixed race kids now and how their school doesn't respect him as a father figure because he is not the same race as his children. He wasn't British by birth nor had it seemed as though he had ever really worked or contributed to the British healthcare system but he ranted about the lack of benefits he receives and the idiocy of all doctors and hospitals here. His disease was mild and his knowledge limited (though he would have vehemently disagreed on both) – I had no use for him and just wanted him to stop talking. I wanted to hear from the other people sat bored around the table – what was their disease like? How were they coping? What were they taking? What was working and what was not?

It carried on like this for a bit (an hour) with a couple of people getting a word in edgewise here and there, but not by much. This guy needed a support group of a very different kind.

Just as I was sat there staring at the loudmouth concentrating every fiber of my being in an attempt at shutting him up through telekinesis another man walked in, a very knowledgeable professor with Sarcoidosis of the lungs and clearly the undisputed leader supreme of this little club of rare disease card holders – and he wasn't having it!

He LOST IT on the guy in a way that really only the truly British can. Told him that all he did was whine and why was he even here then if he was just going to talk on and on about himself. The loudmouth hates prednisolone and refuses to take it, but isn't doing anything else, either- so why was he here? The rest of the group perked up, again alert in their seats and I resisted the urge to applaud the professor.

Then the very British professor told him that if he is as self-absorbed and obstinate at home as he is here then it is no small wonder that his wife of only a year hates him.

The "it's all about me" loudmouth (and professed ninja ex-marine) stood up and the rest of us started backing up nervously from the table, silent and in shock at the exchange. (I was surely the only one in there thinking that this was clearly the most entertaining support group EVER)

As the rest of us were now still seated but a good foot and a half away from the table, just waiting for the loud, obnoxious "ex-military ninja" to leap across the table to actually fight the professor, another woman, who had not yet spoken a word, blurted out that she just "can't believe the gall of the benefits office actually sending someone to check on her" (random?!) and another guy jumped in and said directly to me - I don't think we get nearly enough in benefits for this, how much do you get? I didn't have an answer, I couldn't even process the question as I was staring openly at the professor and the ninja squaring off at each other from either end of the square table, hurling insults and weak retorts. The quiet and elderly chairwoman rose shakily to her feet and passed around cookies, diffusing both the loudmouth ninja and the professor with a chocolate hobnob and calling the meeting back to order.

Oh my God, it was amazing. This group was so full of WIN. So full.

I was so put off by the entire ordeal that it was an entire year before I returned for a second helping of complete and utter crazy. From the forum I had learned that I wasn't the only one scared off by the self-absorbed ex-military ninja. He was even a part of the forum for a while until he eventually left as eventually more people had blocked him than hadn't. I'd not gotten anything constructive out of the support group other than a good laugh in the end, but had been enticed to return with another member, a friend nearby that I had met through the forum as well. She wanted to see this guy with her own eyes and, preparing myself for another dosage of pure crazy fun I agreed to meet her there after work – with drinks following the meeting to decompress.

It was even *better* this time. He was there, again, as he 'never misses a meeting in case someone new comes in need of support and information'. I'd never before met someone who was quite as self-absorbed as this man. In the last year things had gotten worse. His disease was still very mild but he hopped around from doctor to doctor as nobody would give him what he wanted – to be signed off for more benefits. He was now on a campaign to raise awareness of our condition on a national scale – to the point that he bragged about being forcibly removed from the offices of BBC's Channel 4. I challenged him, pointing out that nobody in their right mind would want to make a documentary about a foreign man on British benefits with a mild form of a rare disease – people want to watch something interesting. Something controversial. Something with entertainment value, not a sob story of personal failure.

That did not go over very well.

The loudmouth ex-ninja ranted for a good twenty minutes about how fascinating his life is and how at least he is trying to raise awareness of our condition to the public. He was writing articles, books, writing to papers and going straight to the offices of the BBC. All I could think was please no, don't let this person become the face of our condition. Please please please please no.

His ranting turned again to the lack of love and support from his horrid wife at which point I tuned out and turned again to my phone under the table – only to find that my friend across from me had been sending me silent texts with increasingly elaborate ways in which we could possibly get this guy to stop talking.

The elderly chairwoman (still there!) brought the group's attention to other support groups meeting around the United Kingdom and whether or not we could link with them in any way. The loudmouth ex-ninja jumped in before anyone else could with his great distaste of the 'other groups' which in his opinion weren't really support groups at all. They met in pathetic garden centers and pubs – hardly a proper place for a support group (whereas my friend and I thought that actually sounded very nice!) and *they didn't even have attendance registers!* The horror! What were these people doing, wasting their time and just sat around chatting!

My friend and I left the meeting in a fit of adolescent giggles and headed for a mature support group style drink at the local pub to debrief from the epic crazy that hadn't disappointed.

I'll say one thing about this disease. It sucks, it really, truly does and it has turned my life upside down but holy hell I've also had some of the most entertaining, shocking and amazing experiences with it. If anything at least Sarcoidosis isn't boring.

It's actually been anything but.

My doctor says I'm not a drug addict - now just tap that vein I've got to go!

I love to travel and do so often, though I am never without my issues. When travelling I am the person that obsessively checks for their passport in their bag – even though it is zipped and locked, convinced that it will have leapt out and onto the street at some point during the journey. I will check for my passport in the car before arriving at an airport, then check again before leaving the car *at* the airport. On the walk from the car *to* the airport I will again shove my hand into my bag to frantically feel around for said passport – eyes wide in panic until I feel its rough and well-worn edges. All is right with the world, I can continue to the check in desk – wait, where's my passport?! It was *just* here… oh. It's in my other hand.

When packing I am now of the mantra that if I've got my passport, tickets and bank card everything else is really just a bonus. Since becoming chronically ill, however, "got meds?" has been added to the mantra as I absolutely cannot go anywhere without them. Painkillers, on the other hand, I sometimes forget.

See, I don't really *need* them. Or at least I don't like to need them. I wear patches of painkillers that provide me with a steady stream of relief, so only use the additional painkillers that go with the patches very rarely and only when things are particularly desperate. The two work together, so I am not able to effectively take other types of pain relief. My husband and I have a good laugh about it as my painkillers are all 'black label drugs' and he has to show ID when he picks them up for me at the pharmacy.

Because I like a challenge and being ridiculously diseased isn't quite enough I was at the time also doing a Master's degree at the University of Chester, about a four hour train ride north of London. I was due for a two day seminar and obsessively packed my bag with passport (not sure what for), train tickets (that miraculously stayed in my bag and did not leap out at every given opportunity), bank card, overnight bag and – most importantly – meds. I had enough meds for a week just in case another Icelandic volcano were to erupt and somehow stop British train service.

It is an unfortunate and somewhat humiliating (to me) effect of my medical condition that stress can cause a flare-up of symptoms. I didn't think I was all that stressed – I was actually looking forward to this seminar and to heading up North for a couple of days. Stress, however, can occur with me in something like an aggressive business meeting where negotiations start to break down and I develop sudden Bell's Palsy.

Great party trick, but not all that professional when a business meeting is interrupted by an ambulance and me having to apologize for my newly acquired Texas accent.

Feeling a bit 'off' on the train I arrived, checked in to my hotel, video-chatted with my family and headed off to bed – to wake up at four in the morning with an excruciating, electric pain firing up and down the right side of my face. I leaped out of bed and dove for the meds in my bag, frantically pulling out my med-kit divided in daily drug cocktails and searching for the painkillers. If I could just get them under my tongue and lay back this would pass. I was nearly blinded by

216

the pain, tears pouring down my cheeks and my breath coming out in wracking sobs.

They weren't there. I didn't have any with me. I'd completely forgotten them.

Okay. Okay, okay… okay. How could I get more painkillers in Chester? Now? I'd have to call my doctor as soon as they opened at seven – surely they could fax over an emergency prescription to a local pharmacy, I could get over there and settle down in time for my seminar. I had a plan – I just needed to make it to seven.

For another two hours I laid on the bed clutching cold wet towels to my face and watching hideous early morning television programs about fitness and telephone shopping. The programming gradually switched to family interventions and shows about 'who's the daddy' and seven am gloriously arrived.

It's not necessarily a good thing when you call your GP's practice in the early morning and the receptionist greets you by name, recognizing your voice.

Through sobs I explained my situation and was assured that the doctor would fax over an emergency prescription as soon as she got in – I just needed to give them the details of the closest pharmacy that would have these particular drugs. Spurred on by the promise of progress I found the nearest pharmacy, a Morrison's just across the street from the hotel. I called them, calming myself as best as I could though my voice was shaky and stuttering. I must have sounded like a complete drug addict as I first asked if they *had* these drugs in stock, then asked if my doctor could fax over an emergency prescription and I could come pick them up right now. As it turns out, according to three independent pharmacies in Chester, the drug I needed was a 'black label drug' and could only be given with the original prescription slip, not a faxed copy.

"Even if my doctor called in to explain?"

"Well no, that's just not secure enough. It could be anybody on the phone."

"But you could ask them trick questions about doctor stuff just to be sure!"

Silence.

The last pharmacist at least had some practical advice for me – that I should go to the local hospital, perhaps they could sort me out there. I hadn't even thought of that! I rushed around the room, clutching my cold face towel and shoving things into my bag like I was making a run for it. I made it down the stairs and to the reception, slapping my key on the desk and, through shaking sobs, asked for directions to the nearest hospital. The reception staff were appalled, had I been beaten? Had someone broken into my room? Should they call the police?

Oh no, I assured them with a forced smile, I've just got a 'condition'. That's all. They were about to call me an ambulance when I broke down and asked again for directions to the nearest hospital – the desperation in my voice no longer hidden. Why, it was just across the street – but an ambulance might get here faster.

I barely heard them as I was already half out the door and on my way to the hospital, lurching with my now stiff right leg trailing behind me. Crossing the busy street I looked as though I had just been struck by a car and was just now making my way to the A&E. Two cars slowed to a stop just to look around for what had hit me as I made it to the grass on the other side and speed-lurched across the lawn and to the hospital entrance.

This was not a London hospital. The urgent care center wasn't actually open yet. There was an emergency department, where I first went, but the receptionists were chatting away in a corner making tea and the only other waiting patient was a gentleman quietly snoozing across a few seats in the corner. He may have been the janitor, actually. I stood there, as Canadian as could be and refusing to make a fuss when a wave of pain again overtook me by the face and I let out a screeching sob, gripping the desk for support and eyes blood red from the flare.

I will say this about people in Chester – Northerners are absolutely lovely, caring people. They're not too quick on their feet, though. It took *ages* for the receptionist to make it over to me, looking me over and seemingly more concerned at my foreign accent than physical state. I explained, as best I could in that high-pitched dolphin voice that women take on when they are crying hard, that I had an auto-immune disease, was having an unexpected flare and I was out of my particular painkillers. I was from London, hadn't brought them with me and even though my doctor called the Morrison's pharmacist whose name was Terry he wouldn't give me any painkillers because they are a black label drug and I have a seminar at the university in an hour, I just really need a pack of these drugs to be prescribed so I can go.

The kindly receptionist, having grasped only a small part of my gasping rant, came around the corner and led me to a chair to wait for the urgent care nurse to come in so she could see me, getting me some ice for my face and leaving me there to watch even more horrible daytime TV as the clocked ticked ever closer to the seminar I was about to miss. Couldn't I go in to just see an A&E doctor? There wasn't anybody else here, surely I could explain it to them, get my prescription and go?

No, they said. The proper urgent care team had to get here and assess me first, that's just how things go. I waited, writing around in my chair and clutching my face with all the pressure I could muster. I cried. I tried meditating. I checked the desk again – would the nurse be here soon? Was there any other way?

Although I understood the cause for delay once the urgent care nurse showed up along with two members from the hospital's social work team. Oh my God they thought I was a drug addict.

I was brought into a small room painted a soothing yellow and asked about where I was from, why I was on that drug and why I didn't bring any with me. Did I really need it that urgently – have I talked to anyone about my problems?

Oh no, no no no no no. I didn't have time for this. I needed to get this pain under control so I could get back on with my life – I didn't need a counseling session! Desperate for the menagerie to end I got out my phone and got the phone number of my doctor in London – insisting that the nurse call to confirm that I was *not* a drug addict after a fix and just needed this prescription so I could fix the issue and get on with my day. The nurse reluctantly gave the practice a call, her eyes going wide as the receptionist first assured her of what was happening and then my doctor, who would fax over a prescription to the hospital immediately. The nurse signaled and the social workers left, wishing me well with renewed sympathy at my obvious physical distress. Within minutes I was rushed into the emergency department, seen by a doctor and given not only a shot of morphine in my arm but the painkillers I needed and sent on my way – late for the seminar but still able to make it if I hurried.

Running through the hospital searching for the main entrance I stopped at the volunteer's desk to ask for directions to the university building I was due at – explaining that I was late and asking where I could get a taxi. I'll say another thing about Northerners, they are a *friendly* bunch!

A group of elderly gentlemen at the volunteer desk debated for a moment on the fastest route to the building I needed to get to, determining that it was a mere 10 minute walk and not worth the cost of a taxi (despite my having just been shot up with morphine and shaking on my feet like a leaf) – one spry man knew the way, follow me! he said, he'll show me. Fantastic, I was expecting him to take me to the door and point the way but no, he grabbed me by the elbow and ran me down the hall and *out* the door!

"I know a shortcut Love, we'll go through the parking lot and over the meadow. How late are you and who's your lecturer?"

"What? Um, it started an hour ago and his name is Tony Wallaker – do we really have to run so fast? I'm not feeling great-"

"Oh Tony! Friend of my grandson's! He'll understand that you're late, I'll explain everything. Don't you worry Love, we'll get you there!"

Bewildered I let him run me down the parking lot and into the woods by the elbow, coming out between houses on what I'm quite convinced was private property – a belief reinforced by having to climb over a small fence (It's just to keep the sheep out, he said, not people!) and running over the stones of someone's elaborate front flower garden. We burst out of a hedge onto the grounds of an old building like two convicts on the lam – this was it, he said. Did I know the room number?

222

I thanked him profusely for his kindness, adamantly declining that he walk me right into the classroom as he did exactly that, still leading me by the elbow up the front steps, through the door and following the seminar direction signs posted along the halls. I paused outside the door, still with my elderly handler from the hospital, trying to catch my breath and only then noticing that the pain in my face had finally faded. I listened at the door, whispering another final thanks to my kindly handler as I craned my ears for any sign of an appropriate time to disrupt the group by walking in so late. To my horror the elderly man swung the door open and declared "All right Tony? I found you a straggler at the hospital! She's had a tough morning so go easy on her! All right Miss, I'll be leaving you now – you take care!" to a group of speechless global professionals that had also come in to Chester just for this seminar.

And of course a seat had been saved for me right up at the front.

PET Scan Strap-Down

I seriously cannot be the only one that these things happen to. I just can't. Technicians were running around screaming, I was shouting and trying to squirm out of my restraints...

If you have ever had a PET scan you'll know that it is kind of like an MRI, but for your full body and you are even more squeezed in and strapped down for about 45 minutes in a funky new-age looking type room. Kind of like being in Star Trek. But with narcolepsy. If you've not ever had an MRI before well, then allow me a moment to congratulate you on your good health whilst glowing green with envy.

Anyway, something about the tracer and dye they inject an hour before gives me random yet severe sleepiness and I passed out in my lounge chair clutching my laptop to my chest and snoring like an old man before the nurse had even left the room. My legs went numb but I wasn't even awake enough to let anybody know. I was awake enough to *know* that they had gone numb, but too asleep to do anything about it. I only sort of woke up when the tech came back to remove the IV line but I was so out of it he could have shoved a new IV into my eyeball and I wouldn't have noticed (well, probably). I was woken up an hour or so later by a technician poking me in the side (I was properly asleep) and I shouted at him to 'give me back my laptop' (he didn't have it. I did.) at which he shook his head, recorded my height and told me to go 'wee'.

Odd.

I came out a few minutes later and they were ready for me at the scanner - a lovely woman helped me onto the razor thin star trek bed already positioned halfway through the machine and started to strap me down. This I was not expecting, but fine. What was I going to do, complain? Flail my arms around wildly in my best Braveheart impression? (You can take pictures of my innards, but you can't take my freedom!) Before I could concoct and then make a proper scene my arms were strapped across my chest, my head was strapped to the plastic pillow type thing and even my chin and jaw was strapped into place. I could only move my legs (though I wasn't supposed to) and a large foam wedge was placed under my knees so I could 'relax'. Well, as relaxed as one could be strapped down to a table like Hannibal Lecter and shoved into a tight, loud space.

Thankfully my sudden onset narcolepsy kicked back in with a vengeance and I drifted in and out of consciousness as the bed raised and rhythmically slid in and out of the machine. I wasn't even coherent enough to think of a slew of wildly inappropriate euphemisms as the machine slid me in and out of a large plastic ring at differing speeds and depths. They had put a heavy blue blanket over me as a comforting gesture but it instead served to smother me in a cocoon of heat, sweat and panic. I couldn't move to shift the blanket. They thought I was sleeping (I'm like, the only person that snores through an MRI) so all the technicians had left the room and were having their lunch and chatting away behind their protective glass. - there was no one to call out to so the blanket could be removed. I had to just lay there and take it.

My nose itched. If you have ever been handcuffed (ahem) or put into a strait jacket and your nose itches you may understand that in that moment you cannot think of anything else but the itch on your nose. For about 10 minutes. I even tried to position my lips so I could scratch my nose by blowing upward. I looked ridiculous.

The end came and I could hear the whirring machine start to power down as the bed automatically slid slowly backward, returning to the starting position. Oh thank God, I would be out of the straps soon. Surely they would come and let me out in a minute. My legs were aching from the scan and I was just ready to get out of there and scratch the hell out of my nose. My hair was plastered to my face with sweat from the stupid blanket and I was just done.

The bed was out and it started to lower with a mechanical buzzing sound when suddenly there was another sound - creaking and crunching. Wait, what?! The bed was still going down but it was caught on something - the huge white machine was crunching and rocking toward me as the mechanical bed continued to slowly lower with pre-programmed determination despite the cracking and crunching sound - I tried to get off the bed and out of the way but I was strapped down tight, I raised my legs in the air to get them away from the machine, flinging the wedge into the air and to the side. I struggled out of the chin strap and shouted "Help! Is this supposed to happen?!?!" when the technicians, who had seen the wedge fly past their window, ran into the room shouting at each other to stop the machine manually. Three of them in white had burst into the room like it was on fire. The huge white thing was still rocking and slanting toward me as I frantically struggled against the restraints, legs flailing up in the air at 90 degrees and writhing around with my long legs straight up in the air like an overturned giraffe.

They managed to stop it manually and all stood around me working to get the restraints off so I could get out of there, apologizing profusely and telling me that it was fine, the machine was fine, I was fine, everything was fine. Well what the hell was that then?!

Turns out that they had completely forgotten about the plastic height extender they had put under the bed before I came into the room and it had twisted and bent when the machine slid the bed back into starting position. Scared the living daylights out of all of us.

I felt much more sorry, however, for the wide eyed middle aged man sat in the chair waiting his turn outside when I opened the door, as he had surely heard all of the screaming and running inside. I just looked him in the eye as I passed to collect my things and said:

"make sure you hold on tight."

I couldn't help myself.

Chapter Eight: On Family

Resilience is a rather fun concept in which, when presented with an opportunity, you can choose to dwell or you can choose to continue forward – to learn and to improve. To accept your situation and build upon it, to be defined not by your experiences but by your choices and your journey.

Without my family I would falter, stumble and fall. My husband and children are what keeps me going through this –and they are thankfully always ready and up for another of mum's bizarre adventures.

That being said…

There is the family you choose (spouse, friends), the family you make (children) and the family you get (the *others*). The 'others' are family members in which you really had no choice – it's like a lottery with each family getting variant doses of wonderful and crazy tossed in together like the mystery ingredients of a fridge-raid meatloaf, slightly charred and presented to the world as a complete meal made with love and patience.

Yet only edible if smothered in ketchup and drinking wine.

There is little more in life that I love as much as a good sit down sound-off with people about whose family has more 'crazy'. I also love swapping 'poor stories' (erm, I mean… personal growth challenges?) such as the various uses found as a child for powdered milk and driving around in vehicles that would spontaneously catch fire. My friends all have some fantastic childhood stories and we thankfully have each other to laugh with, having always been able to see the funny side of life. The things that happen to us though, well, you really just couldn't make it up.

Having become ill my mother supported me in her own way which, although not always conventional, worked for us within the relationship we have always had. She would come out with great supportive lines such as 'at least it's not cancer' and 'do you have any idea how badly this is effecting *me*?' More than once she had me crying alone in a hospital room at night after having just berated me for an email I had sent to the family, for something I had said, something I hadn't said…Empathy has never been her strong suit.

Some things that we can take from our childhoods are valuable lessons in how you *don't* want to be. Having a family of your own is an opportunity to re-write your future, to create and instill the ideals that you learned to value – even if you learned these values by watching every family but yours. I learned a lot about the kind of mother and wife that I wanted to be, that I wanted my children to be involved in my life rather than a removed accessory to it. Dealing with an illness was an opportunity to involve my children – I never want to hide this from them to 'spare their feelings' – this is very much a part of their lives as well and we will deal with this as a family, as we will everything in life.

Tearing up at the Eye Hospital

In an attempt to give my husband a much needed break (and to spend a bit more time with my girls on my own), I brought the twins with me to the eye hospital one afternoon. I know, who purposely brings two three year olds to a crowded hospital for an afternoon, how fun, right? Well, I had my reasons.

I walked in for my appointment to an overcrowded waiting room full of patients a good 30 years my senior. Not an empty seat to be seen and certainly nobody else with young kids. Nevertheless, the girls sat there, content in their large double stroller to quietly chat to each other and smile at the people in the room. When they got a bit restless I whipped out their iPads and they literally sat there for hours, munching grapes and playing quietly in the buggy while I sat next to them, jumping up to move the giant stroller whenever someone needed to get by.

Finally my name was called and in we went, buggy and all. The ophthalmologist, a young, friendly woman, had been reading through my very large file and asked me about my eyes, how I was feeling and about my sarcoidosis in general as she hadn't ever experienced a case this severe before. She asked me if there had been any significant changes in my condition or treatment since they had seen me eight months ago.

I told her that I had been hospitalized four times for about ten days each round, about the Bell's Palsy and the scarring in my eyes. I told her about the chemotherapy and the failure of my previous drugs. When she asked about my thyroid and when my blood was last taken I told her about the steroid weight gain and that my blood is tested every two weeks, if not more.

She looked at me with sad eyes and said I had certainly been through the ringer in such a short time. Then I told her about my stroke. She eyed me up and down and commented that it must have been some time ago, I seem so well recovered. I told her it was less than two months ago but that it's fine, I'm fortunate in other ways and we all have to get on with life regardless.

She then looked at the twins and told me that the other doctors and nurses back there had been commenting on them as nobody could believe that two kids of this age had been waiting so patiently, calmly and quietly in the overcrowded waiting room for nearly four hours without making a single fuss. I was of course very proud of the girls and told them so - my kids are wonderful and so sweet. (but the iPads and lack of processed sugar really helps!) She commended me on my upbeat attitude about my health, despite things being so severe and dramatic - all the while taking care of young twins, too - she couldn't imagine how I manage it.

I corrected her that my husband takes care of the girls and I, that this was a rare afternoon that I could have the girls to myself. She was shocked, and asked me why I would bring my children to an appointment like this, knowing that they would be stuck in a waiting room

231

and seeing doctors and things like this if I didn't absolutely have to bring them with me.

I smiled and told her that I'm unfortunately in the hospital a lot and for our family, this is our new normal. I brought the twins because I want them to know that their mum in the hospital is totally fine, and that this is nothing to be afraid of, it's just a small but ever present part of our family, that it's okay. My girls both looked up at me right at that moment and told me that I was okay, and that I was "doing a good job, mum, don't worry."

That poor doctor welled up with tears and excused herself from our cubicle - I could hear her telling our story to her colleagues right then and there who came over to meet the girls and give me a smile. Two nurses even came over with lollies for the girls and chatted with them about their iPad games while my eyes were checked.

I may be a ridiculously unlucky person riddled with faults and disease, but I wouldn't trade my life for anyone else's. I'm fortunate in too many ways to count, and that's what gets me through this.

Like a Playground Hobo

I don't always look the part of a good mother, though, and being diseased doesn't exactly help with that. In fact, it has resulted in some pretty spectacular public parenting failures. Despite my illness I am bound and determined, not always to my own benefit, to be the mother that I always envisioned. I will take them to the park, even if it means draping my diseased carcass over the back of the double pushchair for support. I will take them swimming, even if I am literally dipping my body into an actual cesspool of disease. I will make cupcakes with them, even if the result is something even my Chinese street-dog won't eat and I will push them on the swings until my arms are numb – even if my arms were rather numb to start with that day.

It is never really a good thing when your doctor calls you out of the blue and opens with "We've received the results from your blood test, um… are you feeling okay?"

As it turns out I was severely anemic, on top of everything else I had going on. Something about a normal person's iron range being between 50 to 80 and mine was hovering around 8. Single digits are apparently not very good. Could I come in to see them? Well, it would have to wait until the next day as I was going to be taking my kids to the park, like an idiot.

And this is how, on one of the hottest and sunniest days of the year I found myself pushing a heavy double pushchair up a ridiculously steep hill while not only diseased but severely anemic. The kids were delighted, so I didn't much mind, but by the time we made it to the park I was absolutely heaving and covered in sweat, panting like a wounded, asthmatic hippopotamus. The kids ran for the playground while I attempted to gather myself – muffling my coughing as much as I could. I couldn't stop coughing, it had become a loud incessant bark. At least in a restaurant I could have discreetly escaped to the washroom to cough, choke and die alone but here – in the middle of a playground? I couldn't even hide behind a tree lest I lose sight of my children and a pedophile in a white van snatch them up. So I coughed – and coughed, until I really did start to choke on it. The other mums at the playground had already given me a wide berth – I was the strange coughing woman pacing in the corner of the playground without any kids (they had found the slide and completely abandoned me). The choking was becoming severe – I couldn't take a full breath, panic was starting to set in. I coughed and choked loudly some more, though still trying to conceal the severity of what was happening out of fear of 'making a fuss'. I kept an eye on the children as I moved closer to the fence just in case I needed to give myself the Heimlich maneuver at a children's playground.

The other mothers had started to gather, not yet close (as I was still the strange coughing woman without any children at a playground) but watching and waiting to see what would happen. I choked and coughed harder, trying to dislodge whatever was choking me, my neck bobbing forward and back with each hack like a panicking chicken. It was humiliating and so loud – it couldn't possibly get worse.

And then I finally coughed so hard that I fell to my knees and threw up all over a children's playground. Women screamed and my children finally, (finally!) came running to my aid. The other mothers rushed over asking me if I was alright and telling me that someone had already called an ambulance, just in case, and it was on its way now.

I have never moved so quickly in my life. The thought of drawing even *more* attention to myself, let alone the playground sick and the thought of how I would even get the double pushchair into the back of an ambulance was too much for me. I grabbed my twins like I was stealing them and bolted for the pushchair – now pulling deep, full breaths of cold air that I had quite possibly just coughed up some problem lymph nodes. I threw the twins into their buggy, completely ignoring their pleas to stay at the park to see the 'whambulance' and the clear concern of the other mothers. I was out of that playground like a shot, through the anti-pedophile gate and back down into the ravine and toward home, never to return to that particular park ever, ever again.

I was a playground hobo, and it wasn't pretty. Not at all.

Like a pack of sleep ninjas

My family, like most, is an integral part of what keeps me going each day, despite my condition. One of the most difficult aspects to deal with of my condition is debilitating fatigue that is not remedied by sleep – your body is so busy fighting itself that it depletes your energy before your eyes are even opened in the morning. So if you are ridiculously diseased, like me, might I suggest the following:

Get an elderly dog. Preferably one that is also a complete jerk-face, like mine. Even on my very worst days when I want nothing more than to crawl under the covers and disappear, the clickity-clack of that little ingrate tap-dancing off my bed and down the hall to go pee on something is enough for me to leap out of bed like Xena the Warrior Princess and corral that little dog down the stairs and outside. By the time he has maliciously peed on everything I own outside and I let him in, after having stood there swaying on the spot in agony watching him take his sweet time, I am usually feeling much more awake and alert, ready to take on the day.

I like to set my alarm clock to the top-40 music station that all the kids are listening to, Capital FM, not anything good. If it were good it would be likely that I would drift off again, content and happy. This is unacceptable for diseased persons in the morning. Capital FM is pretty much guaranteed to play a God-awful Miley Cyrus song once every six minutes and if the crappy music doesn't get you out of the bed and awake the memories and visions of her musical performances involving foam fingers on stage will have you wide awake and horrified in no time.

Try having young children, preferably twins. Every morning my three year olds come padding into our room for a family cuddle which, in itself, would be quite lovely – but the previously mentioned shih-tsu is usually in there under the blankets (spooning me, completely inappropriate) and, given that for years my husband's favorite household game to play with the dog was 'bedsnake attacks' – in which the dog believes he is being attacked by Satan from his hiding place under the covers and proceeds to lose his brain in a frantic biting and barking frenzy. Diseased exhaustion or not there is nothing quite like a shih-tsu chomping your bum cheek first thing in the morning to really wake a person up.

True love brings not flowers but an iPhone charger

Oh the holiday joy of being ridiculously immunosuppressed - as I've landed in the hospital again, this time with pink eye.

Laugh away, I was horrified and all of my fears of hypochondria raised up in full force. I had a particularly violent flare the day before, waking up in the morning having to claw my left eye open as it had swollen shut.

It was the reaction of my husband, however, that reminded me of what a charmed life I do lead, despite these little 'hiccups'.

I called my doctor early on in the morning to ask whether I should go to the practice or straight to a hospital (I never know any more) and was told to come in straight away, she will take a look. Now, when your well-seasoned GP's reaction upon you walking through her door is "Holy Hell!" it is very rarely a good sign.

I was given some antibiotic drops and sent straight to the hospital as "my case is too complicated to be handled in the community". I got back to the car where my husband and children were watching youtube videos of My Little Pony and was told off by two irate three year olds for interrupting the plight of Twilight Sparkle. I told my husband that I couldn't go to the hospital as I only had 27% battery on my iPhone and had left my charger at work the night before - maybe I should just go to the office instead. Oh god, now it was at 24% - how could it drop so fast?!?

Oh no. He wasn't having that. As he drove me to the hospital he suggested that I close some apps to save power, but I had just updated the phone and had no idea how to close apps now. Plus, googling it would take unnecessary battery and I needed to save that precious 27% for vital communication processes like Facebook, checking work emails and texting my friends like an obsessive teenager.

Prince Charming that he is he dropped me off outside of the A&E, told me to call him to come to get me as long as it isn't during rush hour and he hurried away to get the kids off to school as I walked in, horrified at having to explain that I was there for pink eye.

I was brought in and quickly admitted once the severity of my immunosuppression came to light, though this still took a number of x-rays, blood and neurological testing over the span of a few hours. My phone battery was becoming a major point of stress, people wouldn't stop texting me - didn't they realise how much power they were taking?!? How was I to let my husband know that I was alright, what was happening and when to come get me? By the time I was wheeled up to a ward (I really wish they would just let you walk. Sitting in a wheelchair from an eye injury is humiliating enough, but being wheeled through the hospital Hallway of Shame with everyone staring at your swollen eye and perfectly fine legs in a wheelchair is just too much) my phone battery had reached a critical level of 2%. It was going to die at any time. I had to turn it off completely to save that precious 2% for when I needed it. Turning it off (even the iPhone wasn't cool with this. It asked me if I was sure three times) I zipped the phone into my bag, promising myself that I would only turn it on to call my husband when the time came.

So there I was, sat in my bed on the ward panicking that I couldn't tell my husband where I was. I considered going down to the hospital shop to buy a bottle of water so I could get cash, then buy something else so I could get change and then use that to call him from a pay-phone. Do they still have pay-phones? They must, those famous red London phone boxes can't be empty, surely. But do they have one in the hospital? What to do, what to do! And what if the hospital shop doesn't give cash back? WHO USES CASH OR COINS NOW ANYWAY?!?

My kindly Ecuadorian roommate pulled out her phone - an iPhone! The heavens opened and the angels sang, an iPhone! I calmly and politely asked her in a combination of my high-school Spanish (I even managed at one point to actually ask her *Donde esta el baño*? and meant it) and charades if she had a charger - and she did! Yes! I refrained from leaping over there and dancing in glee to collect this poor woman's charger only to find that she had an iPhone 4.

Damn.

I won't lie, I actually burst into tears, and with my eye the way it was that was exquisitely painful. I was so desperate to contact my husband to let him know that I was okay and was admitted but probably being sent over to the Western Eye Hospital shortly. I would have to sneak down to the shop to try my pay phone plan when the woman kindly offered me her phone so that I could send my husband a text. A angel among us, this woman was, and I held her phone with the utmost reverence as I typed out a short message to my husband of where I was and where I was going, could he meet me there? It was ready, I just needed to enter the phone number to send it to and everything would be fine.

What was his phone number again? It is saved into my phone. I don't think I had ever had to actually dial it before. 07867...07876...07856. I could have cried. I was so close. I was holding a working phone and the text was right there waiting to be sent - and I blanked on the number.

Even worse, I didn't know ANYONE's number. Except my office, and they were closed. Even so, would they even have his number? I couldn't call my house phone as I don't have that number either. Phone books are dead and would his mobile even be on one online? I realised then that even if I had miraculously conjured up appropriate coins and found an antique pay phone that I would have no number to call. The only thing I could think of was to find A LOT of coins and call my father in law, sleeping in Canada, and to have him call my husband for me to relay a message. I couldn't call an overseas number from this woman's phone, that would have been far too rude. What was I going to do? I was so close! And why has no one yet invented Facebook stands to replace outdated pay-phone locations? Just a touch screen with internet access for coins or even better, scanning your bank card. Someone should really get on that.

I sent the text to my best approximation of my husband's phone number (he never got it) and prayed that it was the right one (being an atheist I had little hope in this plan but was desperate enough to try anyway). It was sent. I had done the best I could and I was quite certain that I had texted my message to the right number, so I sat back onto my raised hospital bed and had a little nap.

I woke to a team of doctors around my bed debating the look of my swollen eye in terms of my impending chemotherapy on Friday, and they suggested that they keep me in hospital for the week until an Ophthalmologist can come to see me, perhaps we could do the chemo infusion here?

Oh hell no. I was adamant that I would be going home that evening, and assured them that if they called ahead to the eye hospital I didn't mind going there on my own. After much back and forth it was agreed that I would be discharged, go to the eye hospital and if they chose to admit me that was the end of my options - otherwise I could go home, provided that I kept my eye bandaged for the trip like a pirate. Again.

The complete loss of depth perception while wearing an eye patch is an experience in fun all of its own. I walked into two walls and nearly fell down the stairs, smashed a basket of bananas off a shelf while trying to select one and waved my debit card at a cashier in what was apparently a very threatening manner. I may as well have thrust the edge toward his jugular screaming "I will CUT you!" for the look he gave me. A receptionist on her way home took pity on me and called me a taxi with her office phone, then directing me toward the chairs to sit and wait.

Now, you wouldn't think that wearing an eye patch could affect your hearing but it somehow does. The driver resorted to holding my hand and guiding me out of the hospital and into his car like a roofied Helen Keller with the ominous comment "I remember you from somewhere". Oh please, don't kill me and harvest my kidneys, I thought. It has already been a crappy enough day and I have no phone to send out secret 999 messages from the back of the car if this goes south.

I was brought without further incident to the Western Eye Hospital where I sat, depressed and blind in the waiting room for a couple of hours before being triaged and brought into a quiet, dark hallway to wait in peace and away from the cesspool of disease emitted from other patients. And so I waited. And waited. And wondered if my husband had received my message. I wondered if I could find a pay phone here? How shall I get home? Does he know I am okay? Does he care? Perhaps he is just busy with the kids and is just expecting me to walk through the door at any moment.

And so I sat there, waiting and feeling quite sorry for myself and dreading the train home in the cold rain when a nurse came up to me, asking my name - my husband was on the phone and he sounded quite desperate - could I please call him back?

I burst into tears as I told her that I couldn't, my phone had died hours ago and I wasn't able to call him at all as I didn't even have his number - but she did! She had taken down his number! She gave me a conspiratory glance from head to toe and quietly offered me the use of her desk phone, as long as I wasn't long and kept it very brief. In great gratitude I thanked her profusely and followed her to use the phone, calling my husband and still too distraught to properly speak.

It was like a dolphin on the phone. I just heard his voice and burst into that high-pitched blubbering wail of tones that only dogs and dolphins can properly hear. I burst into a desperate wail of "how-did-you-find-me-I'm-having-the-worst-day-I-can't-believe-you-found-me" while my husband, sane but relieved on the other end, quickly told me that after not having heard from me for hours and fearing that I had been mugged and murdered on my way home he had left the kids with his "man flu ridden" mother and drove along the tube line searching for me. He came to the first hospital and followed my path from A&E to X-ray to Rheumatology to the ward I was on and was told that I had been sent on my way to the Eye Hospital - where he sat in the parked car and called every single number he could be put through to for the eye hospital until he found someone who had heard not of me, but the "nice and probably overly apologetic Canadian lady with an eye patch". A nurse recognized me, found this other nurse and she found me and it would all be okay, he was on his way!

I replaced the phone ear piece with great care and thanks to the nurse who was stood by, wringing her hands and grinning at my story and the plight of my husband to find me as she then guided me back to my seat in the lonely darkened hallway to wait, until my name was called for a final round of eye examinations, which included turning my swollen eyelid inside out and swabbing it - a terribly painful process in which I had a very hard time keeping my cool. I hung on to the bottom of the table as a low whine escaped my mouth rising in pitch until I could barely handle the pain of what was being done to my eye when my husband strode right through the door, to my side and silently took my hand.

And he'd brought my iPhone charger.

Over-eager Mommy rides again

My family puts up with a lot when it comes to me. Thankfully, my twin daughters are being raised to think that these types of things are perfectly normal, every family has a neurotic weirdo for a mother, right? No?

I like to think of this book as a set of background notes for their future therapists.

I've always been an impulsive person – such as just up and moving to China when I was 20 on a whim. Or making street critter adoption decisions based on whether or not I could scoop them up and put them into my coat without anyone noticing. Steroids somehow make my already impulsive behavior so much worse. *So* much worse. Upon receiving steroid infusions every couple of months I've been known to make impulse purchases such as a rather expensive new living room set within an hour of being released from the ward and having booked tickets for the family for a Norwegian weekend extravaganza to see Fjords, not having actually looked up what a Fjord was until after I had booked. After having had my steroids adjusted last week I then spent three days trying to convince my husband that we needed to buy a canoe. Right now. I'd even worked out how we would strap it to the car for driving around London – despite no need for a canoe in London. But we *might* go to Scotland and everybody knows that you need to bring your own canoe if you go to Scotland.

Being chronically ill has instilled in me a purpose to get out and live as much as I can, to build the family memories I want for our little team of four. I work full time and don't want to waste the precious few weekends we have as a family – so we get out and do stuff, even if it means dragging my husband and children out and about.

Last summer was the 'summer of camping' (I like themes). We bought our camping kit online – got everything we needed for a typical Canadian style camping trip and proceeded to go camping. Every weekend of the summer. It poured on us like a monsoon – didn't stop me. These were memories we were building! I'd spend the entire summer before either in the hospital or too sick to venture outside – we were making up for lost time. Even if it meant camping in the rain. On one particularly feisty trip we had gone from the hospital for a chemo infusion to Dover to catch the ferry to France for the start of a two week European camping trip – and it was fantastic in every way.

So this year is the 'year of the bikes *with* camping'. We're ready for a cross-over of adventure. The only problem? Our kids are only three years old, and can barely ride their bikes. Too big for the old double bike trailer, too slow on training wheels. Something had to be done.

A bit of googling and the recommendation of a good friend and we had ordered trailer bars off the internet (what could go wrong?). Other than a bit of actual child endangerment, multiple injuries and near-divorce we've found that these things are actually pretty great. You simply hook your toddler's bike up to your bike and tow them along. Perfectly safe and looks very cool. Actually, you look like a pretty awesome parent riding around with your kid gleefully riding along behind you – until you turn a corner along the gate of the busy playground and plow your toddler face-first right into the fence. Cue screaming child and every single person in the park turning to stare, judging you on the cool contraption that just nearly murdered your own child.

I ran over to pick her up, brush her off and have a laugh with my screaming kiddo as falling isn't that big of a deal (although I admit that being mashed into a fence on your bike by your oblivious mother is probably a little bit different) as my husband and other child turned back gracefully and came back with admonishments of 'you need to turn wide, like you're pulling a trailer.'

Thanks, tips.

Okay, brush it off. Walk it off. We're good. I talked Kaitie into getting back onto her bike, though she looked dubious. I promised to go slowly and to stay away from fences. She climbed back on – at which point we then had to have a talk about keeping her hands off the brakes while we are moving. More promises from mum to go slowly and stay away from fences.

Off we went, following my husband and Lochie until a sudden scream and a dragging sound was heard from behind. We looked back to see the toddler bike twisted onto the ground and Kaitie sticking out of a large bush a couple of feet away. Had she jumped? Flown? Leapt off like a deluded superhero? More well-intended comments from my husband of 'turn wide' (we were on a straight path) and 'tell her not to use her brake'. I wasn't sure that her touching the brake could do *that,* but hey, what did I know?

I fished the poor kid out of the bush, lovingly picked brambles out of her hair and bribed her back onto her bike with promises of watching a Disney movie when we got home. She looked at the bike with great mistrust. She wanted more. We were in a crowded park and everyone had just seen my child fly off this contraption face first into inanimate objects twice now – I needed her to get back on the bike and show everyone what a good parent I was, I had very few bargaining chips here. I conceded, and whispered that if she got back on the bike and rode home she could have an ice-lolly while watching a Disney movie. She could even eat her ice-lolly *on the new couch.*

That got her on, though she remained dubious. We did well, feeling a bit of success while riding along behind my husband and Lochie until we had to go through another gate and wham! Mashed toddler *again*! I was going slowly and carefully through the gate – as straight as possible. How in the world was this happening!? We just needed to get home – we were just a street or so away. No more bribery, I resorted to straight-up threats and she got back on the devil-bike. I had convinced her that if she just gripped the handlebars and held on for dear life she would be just fine – and she was, all the way home.

This led me to assume that the problem wasn't *me*, it was fences and gates. And also maybe bushes. Surely if we just went somewhere more open it would be fine.

My husband wasn't sure. He wanted to go back to the same nearby park the next day to do some more 'test runs', as maybe it was a problem with the bike or the bar. Nope, no way was I going back to the same park to publicly endanger and injure my child again. We would have to, at the very least, go somewhere nobody knew us. Another town, maybe? Something more open, without fences and gates? So we drove around for two hours on the nicest day of the year so far trying to find a wide open field with a bike path – which did not exist. We pulled over by a park bench to both google Middlesex Bike Trails on our phones for somewhere to try, oblivious to the two teenagers making out on the bench beside our car. The twins piped up from the back seat with a running commentary of what the teenagers were doing with and to each other until it became so awkward and bizarre that we quickly put the first link's coordinates into the GPS and peeled away – my husband shouting "Awkward!" out the window to the now very explicit teens on the bench as we did.

We ended up in a lovely woodland full of bike trails and people out enjoying the spring day with their own bikes, dogs, buggies and scooters. They all stared and even some took pictures as we set up our matching tandem bike trailers – eager to see how these worked.

I prayed there would be no fences.

A particularly wonderful thing about toddlers is their ability to completely forget the events of the day before – a great benefit at the moment as both excitedly climbed onto their bikes – ready for a ride. We were off and the crowd was impressed. Oohs and aahs were abundant as we rode out of the parking lot, down the path and into the woods… and into a tree.

What the hell was *with* this thing? And why weren't Paul and Lochie having the same kind of trouble? This was supposed to be the 'summer of biking and camping' – how could it be going so horribly wrong already? There were Paul and Lochie cycling away like a couple of graceful swans, hair blowing in the wind and looking like they were in a commercial for family holidays and here was me, unwrapping Kaitie from a tree and brushing mud off her jeans. I stood the bikes back up, assuring passersby that we were fine and that Kaitie wasn't really begging to go home, she's a real kidder that one. I looked at the bar. It seemed fine. It was a bar, what could really go wrong as long as it was still straight? Her bike seemed a bit twisted but I just gave it a good pull and it straightened out alright. Now to get her back on…

This time wasn't so bad, her helmet and vest had taken the brunt of the tree impact and she was ready to try again, given that I promised to go very, very slowly. And so I did, nearly so slow that it was difficult to keep the bike upright, but she was happy and seemed to finally be enjoying herself. I sped up, just a little, anxious to catch up to Paul and Lochie, as well as to get this bike ride properly underway. And so we went, passing impressed looking other cyclists and walking families until out of nowhere there was another screech from behind and a dragging sound – the bike was on the ground *again* behind me and Katie was lying on the ground, traumatized. I was starting to get really upset at this point. I was sick, and was finally feeling well enough to do something fun with the family and it was just turning into a spectacle of being a horrible, abusive mother. My face flushed with shame as I again ran back to collect my crying toddler, with Paul and Lochie gracefully turning back to 'help'. He assured me that it wasn't my fault, something was probably wrong with the bike. We tried switching kids but Lochie shook her head – no way was she getting on mum's deathtrap bike. Kaitie had nearly perfected the tuck and roll maneuver – it would probably be best for her to just stick with it, but this time I would go in front so Paul could possibly see what the problem was.

A bit more cuddles and assurances (straight up lies) and Kaitie was back on her bike and ready to go, slowly. Off we went, in a straight line very slowly. We came to a place where the path veered dangerously close to the river (of course!) and I told Kaitie to hang on tight as I slowly and carefully rode along the path until more screams were heard from behind – Paul yelling for me to stop and Kaitie yelling not so much for me but this time *at* me as she rolled along the path and toward the river, stopping just before going over the short bank, only to be accosted by an over-excited and soaking wet Labrador Retriever. I again leapt off the bike and ran to Kaitie's aid, though she made it very clear that she wanted Daddy, not Mummy. Mummy was far too dangerous.

Heartbroken I turned away to collect the bikes when Paul came to my side, assuring me again that it wasn't my fault – he could see that the bar was twisted. I exploded (steroids didn't help the instant rage) and vented to the world that I knew it wasn't my fault, I knew I wasn't doing anything wrong but poor Kaitie kept flying off that thing and getting hurt. I was feeling like the absolute worst mother in the world as what I had originally intended as a charming family bike adventure had become Kaitie's experience as a crash test dummy. In public.

We decided to remove the bars and let the girls ride back themselves, which they didn't as they were now too terrified of their own bikes as well, given the scene that Lochie had just witnessed. We were about half way back to the car when Paul looked quizzically at Kaitie's bike and the bar hitch on the front. He turned to me and said: "You know what? I think I know what the problem is. I think the hitch is on crooked, and I didn't tighten it enough. No wonder it kept dumping her over."

It wasn't my fault after all.

It was *his*.

Chapter Nine: Chemo Adventures

You busy tomorrow? No? How about some Chemo!

You know that whole "whatever, I'll do anything it takes to feel better" feeling?

I had been struggling with flares over the last few months and had reached a point, while at work, that I just couldn't do it any more. I couldn't take it. My eyes would randomly blur and flare in pain – I was having to keep one dilated to relieve pain nearly constantly, resulting in looking like a hyped-up squirrel. Funny yes, but not particularly professional. In any business meeting it was at least a pretty good ice breaker, when I would shake hands with someone upon meeting them, make eye contact and they would let go and jump back with a "WHOA, *what* is wrong with your eye?!?" See, I run a Chinese company and it's kind of a direct culture. Large doses of steroid infusions tend to give me teenage-like acne along my jaw and I've been asked numerous times, by both my staff and strangers "what is wrong with your face?" My demeanor and appearance were getting to be a bit much around the office.

I was spending my days either miserable at home layered in ice packs and exhausted or at work, layered in frozen peas and napping on a couch the company had brought in just for me. I had reached a level of desperation and couldn't continue like this for much longer. Brain fog – the feeling that you just cannot think clearly and as though your IQ is lowering by the day, had taken over my life. I was forgetting things and had the attention span of a brain damaged golden retriever. I was limping and would have moments in the morning where my husband would put painkillers in my mouth for me as my elbows had swollen too much to bend. I'd tried holding a pill up in the air and dropping it into my open mouth but more often than not it would bounce off my face and be eaten by the dog before I could grab it. Nothing can kill that shih tsu.

I'd had enough, we had to move to another treatment, I just couldn't live this way any longer.

My employer made an appointment that evening for me to see my specialist privately again and, knowing what an emotional and mental mess I was, he arranged to come with me. This doctor had to know how things really were for me (and for the company?) and that we needed to up our game. My company was willing to pay out of pocket for experimental treatment, anything, just to get me back on my feet. Something had to happen, and this doctor could maybe, just maybe, fix me.

Now, there is something about your Chinese employer being willing to pay for experimental drugs for your relatively unknown disease that is somewhat alarming – not least the concept of indentured Chinese slavery to which I was already well embroiled – but hey. Like I said, we were desperate and something had to give.

So on a cloudy Thursday evening at five o'clock my boss, DK, and I arrived at the poshest office (erm… I mean, hospital?) either of us had ever seen. Portland Place, central London. Beautiful entrance with high ceilings, a full coffee bar in reception, a small waiting room full of smart black leather armchairs, soft lighting and modelesque receptionists striding over to take care of our every need. Could I please fill in this paperwork? Would I prefer coffee or tea? Biscuit? Swedish scalp massage while you wait? There wasn't a television blaring mundane re-runs of non-offensive shows – instead the walls were covered in art and the tables were strewn with fresh copies of The Economist and magazines boasting elegant home décor. I waited for no more than a few moments before my name was called and I looked up to find that my specialist had come to reception to collect me himself, smiling and calm. So different from the rushed and crowded atmosphere of the regular rheumatology ward. I can see why they do private work now - I certainly would!

We were ushered in to a large office with high backed leather armchairs and a private examination area in the back. High windows and a soft carpet gave the room a feel of more of an old library than a doctor's office – a complete change from the mass clinical setting of the medical offices I usually frequented.

That, and you know that any doctor's office with a 'complimentary umbrella stand' outside the ornate entryway is going to be good.

DK had come for moral support and to ensure that I was truly getting the best care possible at a schedule that met our own and I walked in confident and holding a list I'd made of issues and questions. I was ready – I was going to be my own best advocate and he was going to listen and I was going to come out of there with results, dammit! Real results! Roar!

I burst into tears.

I told the doctor about the stroke and gave him my discharge papers, as well as foot-long list of my current meds and other letters that he has seen before - reminding him of my case and assuming he had forgotten based on our previous three minute long appointments within the dingy hospital basement. He briefly examined me and declared that the stroke changed things considerably - that Infliximab/Remicade would no longer suffice for Sarcoidosis of this severity - we are going to move on to a different drug-cyclophosphamide - a chemotherapy infusion given once a month. For how long? We'll see. At least six months, probably 12 and then we will try to wean you down onto Remicade (a biological drug not yet approved for use in my condition).

That's about when I really lost it and started bawling like a complete lunatic in his office. I just couldn't keep it together. Gratitude, relief, fear, confusion, frustration - and now so many questions. Chemotherapy was never on the table before, I had never even heard of it being a treatment option. I thought Remicade was the silver bullet and I was just aiming for THAT. When would I get it? For how long? What will happen? How does it work? Do I change my other meds? What's the monitoring process? Are there case studies I can read? Anecdotal evidence about some guy in Iceland 17 years ago that did this and lived? Anything? *Anything?!*

Don't worry, he says. It will be fine, he says. We will take care of you, he says. Go home, calm down, relax and you'll get a call from the registrar soon booking you in for an appointment as soon as possible.

Wait! How soon? Who is this registrar? Do I need to call them? Do they have my number? When will they call? Soon, he says. Relax.

Again with the cue to leave, you ridiculous time wasting hypochondriac. So I did.

I hadn't even made it back to the car (or managed to stop my hiccupping sobs) before my mobile rang - it was the registrar from the public hospital - how far do I live from the hospital and am I free tomorrow morning for my first treatment?

Wait, what?!

It was already after hours so the Registrar told me that she will fill in all of my paperwork first thing in the morning and try to get me booked in, wait for a call in the morning before I start making my way over there, just in case.

Okayyyyy.....?

So I headed home and spent the rest of the evening shell-shocked and frantically googling this new drug - directly against the advice of my doctor to "relax" and "don't google it, you'll just scare yourself". (He was right. Rats). My husband and kids were ill that night and by the time I got home all three of them were already in bed. I didn't have anybody to talk to – I didn't want to wake up Paul. I didn't want to call anyone – I just sat in my puffy armchair and clutched my little shih tsu to my chest for dear life and just stared at my phone – waiting. Chemo. And so suddenly. This was really happening.

I'd like to imagine that people generally get more time between finding out and actually doing this – time to process and freak out appropriately. Thinking back now I can't really see the point – sure it was a bit hectic and stressful but me flipping out about it and pacing the room in a tangent of 'what if's' and worst case scenarios wouldn't have done anything to actually change the outcome. Morning was coming whether I was ready or not. And isn't this what I wanted? Progress? Aggressive treatment? Now?

It just all seemed a bit... surreal. Like it was happening to someone else and I was just there to enjoy the show.

The next morning I was just hanging out with my girls, letting Paul sleep in a bit and charging my phone for the possible call when all at once the loud neighbor came over with something, the dog lost his brain at seeing the neighbor, the girls started fighting and the hospital called my phone. Why? Why God why does everything always come barreling at once? Over the chaos swirling throughout my living room the hospital registrar asked me how long it would take me to get there - an hour and a half if I was pushing it - she said that I had to get there by 10:30 (an hour!) or they couldn't do it today and would have to bring me in as an in-patient next week.

Next week?!

I assured her in my loudest possible voice that I would be there in an hour, hung up the phone and yelled for Paul - he came rushing down the stairs as I ran rushing up, I think the neighbor let herself out and I was a whirlwind of throwing on my clothes and brushing my teeth while Paul called a local taxi company and checked the tube route online to see which would be faster - the taxi said they could get me there in 45 minutes so they won- they were on their way. I ran down the stairs, took my meds, threw on my shoes, Paul tossed me my bag, some cash and my phone and I was out the door and off to chemo in less than six minutes - sweating like crazy and panting- laid out, wide-eyed and hyped up in the back seat of a minicab like I'd just beaten back a werewolf.

Now was not the time to be driving Miss Daisy. I explained the situation to the driver, that I needed to be at the hospital in Central London in less than an hour or I'd miss my chemo infusion – he took off like a bat out of hell, darting through side streets and down the freeway like a maniac on a mission, all the while listening to "Do you really want to hurt me" by Culture Club on Heart Radio. I was posting status updates on Facebook to my enthralled friends of my James Bond-esque race through London to the hospital on a countdown as they were checking and advising me on traffic updates and road closures – the whole thing was just… so me.

Paul then called me so we could talk about what was going on over the phone on my way there - he was arranging for the kids to spend the day at a friend's house so he could come and meet me at the hospital - we hadn't even talked about everything yet! We'd barely talked about anything at all. His advice to me was to just get there, go with it and he'll meet me there, I'll be just fine.

And I was. We made it with mere minutes to spare as I leaped out of the taxi in front of the hospital and zombie-lurched as best as I could to the elevators and up to the immunology day ward where once I got to reception I was grey, sweating and panting too hard to speak. The receptionist looked alarmed and said "Are you Candace?" I nodded while gripping the desk for support and just let them take care of everything from there.

By the time Paul got there all of my tests were done, my cannula was in and I was sat back in a comfy lounge chair playing with my iPad and waiting for the pre-drugs (anti-poison, how comforting) to kick in, cool as a cucumber. No worries – I've got this.

It is strange to have a condition so rare that there is little in the way of anecdotal experiences that can be found online. I had no idea how it would affect me so kind of just went with whatever came. The morning after I felt as though I'd been hit by a truck and well, the nausea was certainly invigorating. I also spent the morning looking at "short hairstyles for large, round-faced people" online.

It kept re-directing me to websites like *www.peopleofwalmart.com*.

I LOVE Chemo!

I'm going to go out on a limb and bet that you don't hear that too often. It is a strange feeling, but amazing to be handed your life back like this. After only two infusions I now spend my weekends at the sea side, taking the kids to a carnival (oh yeah- I am ALL OVER that bouncy castle), going swimming and exploring old castle ruins, walks around the local lake and pub dinners. We go hiking nearly every weekend now. Just three months of infusions and I've accomplished so much at work and personally, finished the taught portion of my master's degree (only a dissertation left!), submitted an app concept, the first draft of my book is 1/3 finished and, most importantly, I've perfected my homemade whole wheat pizza recipe (I can't eat it, but the family can) Also, my zombie apocalypse green beans and tomato plants are doing very well in my first ever garden.

But I'm off to the hospital again. I'm sat here on the packed tube listening to Bob Marley and adamantly ignoring the flare in my right leg, wrist and foot. Trying to think of how I'm going to talk the nurses into pretending to hold me down for the IV line for a picture. Trying not to think about the coma of exhaustion, fever, flare and hulk-smash rage I'm going to be in until Sunday night again. It's fine. Not that bad. The coma-like sleep makes you forget the weekend, really. And I know that one bad week a month is well worth the three fantastic weeks I now have.

Plus, there's Jell-O in the fridge for when I get home, so there's that.

It's just a strange feeling. I want to run to the IV clinic slapping my vein and shouting "fill 'er up!" But at the same time- I know how much the next two days are going to royally suck and it feels like I'm up for a Darwin Award intentionally signing myself up for that.
But at least there's Jell-O.

I've come to realize that these drugs don't affect my condition like they do most people – when your immune system is the problem it actually feels pretty good to have it beaten down into submission. The problem is the flaring that it triggers the next morning and most of the day. I wake up, without fail, shivering in a pool of sweat and crying in pain – wanting to tear out my own spine for any sort of relief. It feels like the drug is battling my immune system in a heated war for territory – a piece of bone, a joint – my eye socket, a

262

piece of spine, an elbow… in a war that rages for only minutes until I feel as though I couldn't possibly handle any more and then it's gone – the drug has won and my immune system has moved on, weakened, to claim other ground. This continues until it has raged through my body and I emerge, hours later, feeling drunk and delirious, ready to devour the entire contents of my kitchen cupboards.

But like I said, it's totally worth it for three good weeks a month.

The Chair

I've come to understand that there is more or less guaranteed to be a standard of weirdness every time I go for chemo. That's just life (well, mine). Clearly the most delightful incident of chaos was at my second infusion, just when I was starting to feel comfortable and like I was getting the hang of this whole thing.

At the Royal Free Hospital in London the infusion clinic is in a tough to find ward (early morning challenge!) on the second floor in a construction zone (yep). Once you get past the builders and distinct lack of signage you come through to a ward unlike others – it's got a relaxed, friendly vibe to it as soon as you are buzzed though the doors. The halls are dimly lit, the nurses are cheery and relaxed (looking) and the patients are wandering around carrying books and seeming to have most of their wits about them (very unlike previous wards I've been confined to) Off the main hall are darkened, comfortable rooms full of plush green armchairs and big windows with people having staked out their spot, surrounded themselves with books and heavy blankets and a hush is felt over the room. It's like a library but with added IV poles and the rhythmic beeps of various monitors. (though the beeps constantly remind me of an old Jermaine Steward song from the 80's – you don't *have* to-take-your… *clothes off!*)

The chairs are delightful and worth a good hour's entertainment on their own - electric loungers! Fantastic! They go up, down, out, in and turn into beds if you want them to. So I kind of set up my little day-camp of my phone, IPad, laptop, chargers, books, fruit and bottled water, kicked off my sneakers and sat back for a day of well, relaxing chemo. There's always that "overly chatty" person in every room, as well as the 'library quiet" people and the one woman with her laptop propped up on the windowsill for the best possible wireless signal so she can obsessively continue to play online bingo.

You learn to tune out everything else and just relax.

And so I did.

I sat back and snoozed, drifting in and out, listening here and there to people coming into the room, checking things, chatting away with niceties and vague interest. The click of the bathroom door, a cough, a yawn…   a snap… a creak…a… thunk? and WHAM I was on the floor.

That chair EXPLODED!

Out of absolutely nowhere the headrest had fallen off the chair as the back panel broke apart – I tumbled backward out of the chair, flinging my arms out and knocking my IV pole to the floor. I landed on my head and lay there, in shock, staring at the ceiling in bewilderment – my limbs tangled around my IV line and my legs sticking straight up in the air, still partially on what was left of my chair. I looked like some kind of twisted up yoga master – and I was stuck. Even worse was that I had not only taken out my own IV pole, I'd completely wiped out the pole of the elderly man sat beside me as well. My tray table had gone flying – having also covered myself, the floor and whatever was left of that chair with water. I hadn't even done anything – I had just been sleeping!

Well, when seven people in a chemo-room suddenly press their Nurse Buzzers frantically at the same time and start yelling for help, people come running. Not just a nurse, a pack of nurses. And doctors. And health care aides. And wanderers from the hallway. And they all stared at me in silence and confusion as they pieced together what must have just happened, a bewildered nurse retrieving a chair arm from across the room. I couldn't even get myself up for fear of dislodging the cannula in my arm. All I could do, as I lay on the floor in a mess of water, wires, cords and chunks of upholstery was to look at the crowd and in my most composed voice say:

"I think there's something wrong with my chair."

Absolutely humiliating.

On the other hand I'm just pleased that nobody ever sent me a bill for it.

The Omen Bird

After everything that had happened on every chemo trip so far, I had every reason to suspect that every possible mishap that could have happened had already occurred and, though cautious, made an early start for chemo round four in an attempt to score the "good chair" at the window. Arriving a full half-hour early I came upon the darkened room of cushy green lounge chairs and made a bee-line for the coveted perfect chair at the very back of the room.

The chair's positioning was ideal in every sense. Sat beside the only window in the room with a view of green, leafy parks and bustling life on the high street below. The bathroom was within easy shuffling distance but far enough to remain fairly immune to the noises coming from within (on a chemo-ward this can get pretty graphic). The chair faced the entrance to the room as well as the hallway – a perfect spot for people watching and shameless eavesdropping. It was, quite clearly, the perfect spot.

And it was mine.

The room filled as the morning wore on, a fleeting look of disappointment flickering across the face of each patient as they came in to settle in a chair, seeing that the perfect spot had been taken. Pleased with my rare good fortune I leaned back, kicked my feet up and gazed out the window, thinking to myself that this must be a good sign, today was going to be a good day.

And then a bird flew right into the window.

A great big, black crow-looking thing. Out of absolutely nowhere it slammed head-first into the window, wings spread wide right toward me. It was although this bird had been aiming for me. I jumped up and screamed, dancing around my chair shuddering with the sense of spiders crawling on my skin. I couldn't even speak I was so freaked out – I just flailed around and made noises. Even worse is that there is a generator of some sort beneath the window, with wire mesh layered high above it to protect the area from falling debris. That wire mesh was right at the level of my window, and now held the lifeless, sinister looking body of this dead bird – exactly at my eye level whilst sitting in the chair.

And it was looking at me. Its neck was twisted and its wings were spread but somehow it was staring straight at me. Like it was *my* fault it flew into the window in the first place.

There were no other chairs, every chair had been taken. I asked aloud if anyone wanted the "window seat" but nobody offered. They had all witnessed the bird flying straight for me and my jumping around screeching like a lunatic. They could all see the dead bird lying there, staring at me with those cold, dead eyes. I was suddenly

267

feeling much less smug about having scored the "good" chair that morning, and settled in for what was by far the creepiest eight consecutive hours of my life, made inexplicably worse once the janitorial staff tried (and failed) to remove it from above with some sort of claw on a stick.

They say that a dead bird represents the loss of freedom, or of freedom coming to an end. A black bird somehow making everything even more sinister. This is not a comforting symbolism when sat in a chair waiting for chemo. Not at all.

And I'm pretty sure that thing was aiming for me.

Fight! Fight! Fight! Fight!

I had to break up a fight with my IV pole.

Seriously.

Since starting my chemotherapy infusions every four weeks I've been feeling pretty awesome for most of the month - with the added benefit (side effect?) that my chemo sessions are so ridiculously entertaining that I have requests from friends to go with me. Not because they're awesome friends and want to hang out with and support me, but because they don't want to miss this level of entertainment.

There was the exploding chair. The dead bird. The big fainting scene with the cannula and the frantic rush to chemo in the first place.

But this one? Even I wasn't expecting something like this.

I went to chemo in the morning as usual, and because I'm on this special diet and because hospital food is pretty awful, I packed my own lunch. No worries. They take my blood, it comes out unusually slowly but I internally blame this on the fact that I've agreed to let a student do it (I'm an idiot) and, after six separate stabbings her supervisor takes over because the poor student can no longer see clearly through her tears. I'm sat there clutching a cardboard vomit bucket for dear life, turning even whiter than usual. Through dry-heaves I assured the poor girl that it was fine, don't worry about it, everyone has to learn at some point. Sometimes I think I'm too Canadian for my own good.

Blood goes off to the lab and I sit back to nap and wait, as usual. (God I love naps. Who doesn't? Weird people, that's who.) I'm woken up a couple of hours later because they for some reason need more blood (I've already given enough to feed a small vampire family for a week) and they send it off to the lab again, apologizing for any delays this might cause. I assure them that it's fine, it isn't like I've got anywhere else to be anyway.

Lunch comes and goes and I eat the super healthful lunch that I packed while everyone else munches on crisps and chocolate bars from the food trolley. I look around with smug contempt, until I realize that even with my healthful meals I'm *still* the fattest person in the room.

Damn.

I continue to sit there, playing on my iPad and getting some work done on my laptop when the fire alarm goes off. Like, an actual alarm, not just a drill. Nurses start running and making calls and prepping old people to be carted outside. Well, this day just got much more interesting! It is determined that we are not to be evacuated (sad trombone) at that moment and for us to just sit tight, the fire has been contained. No worries.

Hours go by, with still nothing having come up for my infusion from the pharmacy. The nurses apologize. Angry little old ladies are starting to really lose their cool - no IV drugs are coming up and we're all just sat there watching the paint dry. Not cool.

A doctor finally comes in to announce that, apologies- the pharmacy was on fire, hence the lack of drugs coming up - the drugs are being brought over from another hospital, hold tight, sorry about that.

This is fine. To me, this is funny as all hell. Of course the pharmacy was on fire. Why wouldn't it be? Until I realized that I would now be stuck there for dinner.

That's about when things really went downhill.

I had nothing. I'd eaten my apple snack and was planning to have dinner at home. I couldn't eat the hospital dinner offered of potato and cheese pie with green pea paste - my dietician would slap me! I had to venture out to forage for food - with my IV pole.

Although the nurses gave me the side-eye, after finally being hooked up to my IV I unplugged myself from the wall and slowly maneuvered my spindly IV pole down the hall and into a queue for the elevator, in which I jokingly asked for directions to the stairs, frightening one poor woman off down the hall and as far away from me as she could get. Well, *I* thought it was funny.

Lo and behold, the cafeteria was closed due to the pharmacy fire. I'm not sure how those two are related, but fine, whatever. There is a coffee shop and a bookstore that sells food (weird) at the main entrance, I could try for that.

Have you ever wandered around a hospital with an IV pole? Not only is it a lot of fun (people give you some fantastic looks of surprise!) but the difficulty in guiding a pole that desperately wants to spin and dance around while you are literally tied to it - also while watching dark blood start to go *up* the IV line and wondering if that's normal or not - is a pretty great way to kill time.

The coffee shop had nothing but pastries, brownies and sandwiches - nothing my "prisoner of war" diet would allow, the bastards. Seriously, how can a hospital not sell healthy or healthful food? I figured I would try the bookstore and hobbled out, vaguely noticing a bit of a kerfuffle going on between two women in the back. I was on the desperate hunt for carrot sticks, my attention could not be diverted.

I did not find carrot sticks at the bookstore.

What I did find, however, was a cold vegetable samosa, a block of cheese and the newest Sophie Kinsella novel - fantastic! All I needed now was a nice warm tea and I could head back upstairs to my chair of despair and misery with my crappy dinner and tea - back to the coffee shop with me!

I get back to the coffee shop just across the hall and notice that a lot more people seem to be hurrying out than going in - and can hear the two women arguing loudly in the back. Something about "God loves you and wants to help you" and the other woman screaming and having a fit that God isn't real and she doesn't want to hear it, how dare you preach at me, blah blah blah. More people got up and quickly left.

I, having nothing better to do, paid for my tea and leaned against the counter, with my IV pole, waiting for my tea and ready to enjoy the show.

It got worse. Much worse.

The disturbed woman started screaming that she was here on being "sectioned" (committed) and didn't need strangers like her preaching at her, and started to pull her own hair. The evangelical woman seemed to have her own wide range of poorly contained crazy and started shouting that God led her to this woman and it was her duty to convert her. You seriously could not make this stuff up. Then the committed woman stood up and started screaming nonsense - prompting the evangelical woman's inner sense of self-preservation to finally kick in as she got up and started backing away. I was still watching the show with my eyebrows nearly in my hairline until I realized -

Oh crap, they were coming toward *me*!

Massive dilemma - I had paid for my tea but the guy was too busy watching this drama to finish making it yet, these crazies were coming toward me and there was nobody else in the shop aside from myself, the kid working the shop and the two crazies getting ever closer and louder. What do you do? Do I get the tea? Back away to the side and hope that the sandwich fridge works as camouflage? Even if I did get my tea in time to run out the stupid IV pole doesn't go that fast....

I stood there like a deer in headlights, not knowing what to do and making small jerky movements in all directions. So basically I stood there and had a "decision seizure" of twitching in any direction my mind was contemplating running to while they came ever closer. I decided to abandon my tea and make a break for the door - they followed me! I was now backed up against a wall, holding onto my IV pole while these two continually bumped into me while pushing and screaming at each other. The committed woman pulled the evangelical's hair. The evangelist slapped the committed woman. My pole was knocked into the wall and there were screams about the power of Jesus and then the committed woman yelling "get away from me" - to *me*!

Oh, that's when I lost it.

I grabbed my IV pole with both hands like the Sword of Damocles and thrust it between them, having lifted it completely off the ground, bags of liquid swinging from one woman to the other and screamed "*I JUST WANT TO GET TO THE DOOR!*"

This was thankfully bizarre enough for both of them to snap out of it and look at me - to which I then got between them, faced the crazy evangelical woman and told her "Yes, God is great. Thank you for the message, but you may have better luck out there" and shoved her toward the door - she wisely took off running. I'm not sure who she was more afraid of - the committed woman or me.

I then turned to the raging committed woman and sympathized "Oh I *know*! People like that are *so* frustrating! I can't *believe* she would just come up and do that to you!" which placated the crazy committed woman to the point that I had gotten her to sit down quietly. Well, quietly muttering to herself which was improvement enough, really.

Adrenaline pumping I then strolled over to the counter, collected my tea from the speechless barista, walked back across the hall to the bookstore and quietly suggested that the bookstore clerk call security.

I then trekked back upstairs to my chair of misery to relax, enjoy my chemo and eat my block of book-shop cheese.

And it was delicious.

Internet Black Hole of Death

It's a strange thing now to be suddenly… disconnected. Professionally I am rather glued to my iPhone with my email, wechat and answering the many calls, texts and emails I get each day. Personally there is Facebook to check, twitter to follow and status updates to post. Various forums full of drama and all of our news is now viewed solely online. Something happens in the world and we know, instantly, and respond.

Take that away from people and you get a very desperate lot.

It never ceases to amaze me how poor mobile and internet reception is in hospitals. Every hospital I have been in has either had some sort of signal blocker, been too close to a prison, had walls too thick or for some, or is a signal dead-zone. An internet black hole of death to which there was no remedy. You would think that hospitals would see happy and engaged patients as easy patients but no – signal is still blocked. These patients have little left to do than to complain, try to chat up nursing staff and wander the halls aimlessly with their mobiles held high in the air trying to get any bars they can. Desperate women hang their phones and laptops out of hospital windows to play online bingo as though it were their only source of income. Business women, like myself, pace the halls asking perfect strangers how many bars they have and what carrier they are with like some sort of new age pick up line. Entire afternoons are

devoted to group rants about O2 and Vodafone –
debating which is least reliable while on a moving train
through the Lake District.

Desperate requests are made to the nursing staff – my
phone doesn't have any bars. Can I use your landline?
Does it go out of the building? Can you make a call to a
mobile from a landline?

"I don't think so" chimes in another patient. "They
don't use landlines anymore."

"Does it connect to the internet?" asks another patient
who has gotten up from her chair and shuffled over to
the nurse's desk to join the crowd. Rumblings and
rumors of a working phone have travelled down the
ranks and other patients are starting to creep over.

"It can't connect to the internet," says the first patient,
"it has wires. Look. They go into the wall." We all grip
our signal-less mobile phones a little more tightly, awed
at the very concept of this large plastic phone attached
to the wall.

"Where does the battery go? Does the power come
from the wall? It's not plugged in to an electrical outlet!
How does it actually *work* then if it hasn't got any
power?"

The nurse eventually lies to us that the phone cannot
dial out of the building and no, we can't just 'have a go
anyway' and the mob slowly shuffles back to their
chairs holding up their mobile phones in what looks to

be a silent tribute to technological progress but is really just another desperate attempt to get more signal bars.

Desperation really starts to set in after about two hours – when so much in the world may have changed and we just wouldn't know. London could be under attack – we wouldn't have a clue. A quiet woman with her phone pressed against the window glass can't take the pressure anymore and bursts out "I have to call my *sister*!" to which other patients nod and agree that our connectivity predicament is grossly unfair and quite possibly a human rights violation that someone should speak to a doctor about.

"Is everything alright with your sister?" I ask, empathetic to her plight. "Why do you need to call her?"

"I just need to call her."

"Is everything alright?"

"I have no idea! I've not been on Facebook for hours!"

I was going to suggest that she try using a payphone down in the lobby but I just didn't think the poor woman would be able to handle it.

I've found that the only way to get any internet action is to shamelessly lie to the nursing staff about where you are going and why. Being a vegetarian I have a reasonable excuse to opt out of the lunch served in favor of trotting down to the cafeteria for something a bit more… healthful… to eat. I tell them that I am a very slow eater (it's the medication, I'm sure) but assure the nursing staff that I will be back as soon as I can and if anything goes wrong with my IV the whole place is full of doctors – what's the worst that could happen?

So I am released and as soon as I am out of their range of sight I bolt through the double doors and down the hall, tempted to lift and carry my IV pole to speed things up. Why, *why* does that thing have to twist around so much when you are in a hurry? I am on a limited window of escapism and I quicken my pace from zombie-lurch to painful-Olympic-speed-walk-that-I-will-regret-later, going straight past the turn off for the cafeteria and toward the front entrance of the hospital, IV pole in tow. It's freezing and dark outside but that matters not, even the drizzle of rain cannot stop me despite the fact that I already have no immune system and the drugs I am connected to greatly increase my chances of getting pneumonia.

I find a spot on the many benches out front amongst the heavy chain smokers – staff, patient and visitor alike and watch my phone with gleeful relief as the top left of the screen fills up with bars. I have a signal! My phone immediately overwhelms me with the pings and dings of incoming texts, messages, chats, emails and calendar notifications and the swoosh of my outbox pouring out the emails I had typed up an hour before. Relief, sweet relief. A feeling of peace and calm pours over my very soul as I read messages and emails, respond and quickly check the news. And an internet forum. Or two.

A smoking nurse came over to me – I guess this is what smokers do? Is it normal to approach strangers and strike up a conversation if you are both smokers? Are smokers just more sociable people? She looked at me kindly as I sat with my knees up around my chest for warmth in my flimsy t-shirt, gripping the frozen metal IV pole in one hand and my phone in the other.

"Smoking is very bad for your health, Love. Especially on *that*" as she points to my bright pink IV bag labeled *Chemotherapy*.

I looked up and smiled. "Oh, God no. I don't smoke. I'm just here for the internet reception."

I can't even get good news like a normal person

Something I hadn't before experienced was the concept of drug funding within the NHS – although my doctors were recommending a certain drug they couldn't just prescribe it as it wasn't yet an approved drug for my disease. This led to funding applications – lengthy processes in which I remained on chemotherapy until a decision was made on whether or not I could have this drug.

I explored pursuing the drug, a monthly infusion, privately but would not be able to sustain a cost of just over £4,000 per month out of pocket without resorting to prostitution and selling organs that I didn't really need.

So I waited.

It was an application that I could do nothing about. I didn't have to provide much information apart from what my medical team had asked of me – nor could I present myself at a decision panel or even write a long sob-story of a letter to persuade key decision makers on what was essentially preserving my life. I couldn't present a business case – despite my adamant view that the cost of this drug was outweighed by the benefit of keeping me fit to work – as I employ nearly fifty people who all pay tax back into the NHS. I was ready to try anything – but my hands were tied.

Each time I arrived at the hospital for an infusion or other test the Rheumatology Registrar, a lovely woman with a wicked sense of humor, would update me on the progress of the funding application – mostly that there wasn't any. Nothing we could do but wait and again, I was happy to do so. She seemed to be more disappointed in the delay than I was and assured me over again of how strong of an application it seemed, we should have a result soon.

New Year's Eve 2013 I was keeled over in bed with food poisoning and no immune system – a nasty combination with my husband so worried that he had my GP on standby. I could barely keep my head up or water down – and then my phone rang, at 7:00pm on the 31st of December – it was the Registrar, and she had great news!

"Wonderful news! Your funding application has come

back and you have been approved!"

"Oh? Wow! That's bleaaaaaaaagh great!"

Pause. "Um, are you alright?"

"Fantastic! I'm just really thrilled!"

"Okay – so we will bring you in this Friday for your first treatment –"

"Bleaaaaaaaaaagh! I'm so sorry about that – yes, Friday. I'll see you then. Thank you so much, I'm so bleaaaaaaaaaaaaagh … excited. I'm so excited."

"Are you sure you are alright?"

"Just food poisoning. Totally fine."

"Umm…Is your head in a toilet?"

Pause.

"…Maybe."

And that is how I rounded off 13 months of chemotherapy for a new drug that could change everything. It's not been easy, but it sure has been fun.

Chapter Ten: On Diseased Travelling

I am an idiot. I not only accept that about myself, but I embrace it. Since having the twins my husband has become a stay-at-home parent and has shined in the role of taking care of not only our daughters but myself, my illness, our finances, our home, our social lives – everything. All I need to do is work. For a while when my illness was raging out of control my husband even got me to and from work – either driving me to tube stations, picking me up at obscure tube stations when I wasn't able to stand to disembark at my stop and even arranging taxis to and from my office. At times he would drive me to work, pick me up and even arrange my medication refills with the pharmacy on the way home. At some points he even knew my own hospital schedule better than I did, delivering me from hospital to hospital and handing me cash as needed.

See, I have become so dependent on my husband that I'm not entirely certain that I can function without him at this point. As a mother I am a complete and utter failure, having never before even purchased diapers for the twins until we experienced a death in the family and my husband caught a flight back to Canada that same night – leaving me with the twins, a full time job and not enough diapers to last the week. I was so pathetic that after day 2 a good friend uprooted herself and her own young son to come and live with me while he was gone – for fear we would all starve and I would burn down the house trying to give the children a bath. I was so helpless that in purchasing groceries online I got the wrong kind of everything and the twins and I survived on takeout food until Janine arrived with her son to save us all. Having purchased pull-up diapers for one year olds this ended in a mess of poop being sling-shot across the room and onto the wall – at which point I burst into tears and called in a cleaning agency.

Being so entirely dependent on my husband has its perks, certainly, but I also tend to wander through life on a cloud of 'it will all work out, I'm sure it's handled' for any matter outside of my career. It is an unfortunate reality that this is rarely the case, however.

The simple matter of calling my bank will put me in tears every single time. To begin, the British automated reception service seems to understand every accent in the world but a Canadian one. Nothing I say registers, until I am baring my teeth at the phone and rapidly pressing zero like I'm sending an angry telegram. Then God help me when I actually get to speak to a person, as the security questions are impossible for someone like me that relies on direct debit and my husband to handle my life. No I do not know the exact price of shoes purchased last month, nor do I recall the name of the store. It was in a mall, does that help? They were black heels. No? Okay, next?

Pass. Pass. Pass. What do you mean I can't 'pass'?

Look. My rent is around this much. It goes to the letting agency. Baker something. No I don't know what day it comes out. Around the middle of the month? I am calling because I cannot access my online account, so how can I possibly look on there to answer your questions? Who memorizes the amount and date of their internet bill? Can I just put my husband on the phone? He runs my life, I don't know these things. Yes, I realize that's not a healthy relationship dynamic. Look, I'm not calling for marital advice, I just want my bank card re-activated.

So calling my bank to check on whether or not my illness is covered by my travel insurance was an entirely new experience in pain and frustration – particularly given that I have a rare disease and not 'just lupus or something' as the insurance advisor would have much preferred. The usual song and dance routine of explaining my condition commenced, with the insurance advisor having to put me on hold to check with the underwriters. The underwriters come back to him with the verdict of 'uninsurable'.

"Not even a little bit insurable?" I ask him, meek and hopeful.

"Well, we can insure your luggage."

Pass.

Finding travel insurance that will not only insure me but also do it for less than the actual cost of the trip has become a social obsession of mine on hospital day wards. I have always been a shameless eavesdropper but now I was a woman on a mission. I now strike up more unsolicited random conversations than my Grandfather in a Walmart. Oh hi, what are you in for? Oh that sounds rough, you poor thing! Have you been able to get away on holiday? Sometimes that can be really helpful in coping. Oh you have? To Spain you say? That sounds lovely! Who did you get your travel insurance with, how much was it and what were the medical questions like? Do you remember the name of your advisor? Hold on, let me get a pen… and then I move on to the next ward for further intelligence gathering.

Oh God. I've become the crazy Chatty McChatterson on the day ward.

It's worth it, however, to continue to live and to do what we love – to bring our distinct following of crazy and adventure abroad, to travel.

Fat-Breaking a ride at Disneyland

We took the twins to Disneyland Paris for their 3rd birthday. For what it's worth, the girls had a fantastic day. They loved everything about it - dressing up in their princess dresses for the parades, Ariel waving at them, seeing Tinker bell and watching Stitch Live.

We didn't go on a lot of rides, though. Mostly due to the average waiting time being an hour and a half each. We did luck out at the Magic Studios and stumbled upon Aladdin's Carpet ride with only a 15 minute line - so we parked the buggies and jumped in line, pleased as peacocks with our rare good fortune.

And then things went downhill.

The ride itself is something like a pretty standard children's ride - four bench seats on each carpet-car that go high up in the air and spin around in a circle, going up and down to the short-lived delight of children and adults alike.

The line took about 20 minutes to get through and once at the gate we scrambled for a carpet to ourselves, Paul and Kaitie in the front with Lochie and I in the back. The lap bar came down, no problems there, the bell went off and the carpets started to rotate around the center of the ride, picking up speed and delighting the girls.

Everyone's carpet went up but ours.

Ours tried to go up, we could feel it shiver and jolt at the effort. But it wasn't going anywhere. Just around and around and around - the only ones on the bottom while everyone else was screeching and flying around up top. Paul turned to look at me, bright red with humiliation and looking at me as if to question what had gone wrong.

We fat-broke a ride at Disneyland.

I started laughing. Like, really laughing. Tears streamed down my face as we whirled round and round along the very bottom of the ride, Paul laughing but trying to shush me so as not to draw more attention to ourselves. I told him to look around, everyone in line and outside of the ride was staring at us - they knew what happened! They knew we fat-broke it! We couldn't possibly draw any more attention to ourselves that wasn't already on us!

Throwing my hands up in the air I shouted "wheeee!!", the girls joining me as we went around on the bottom with our hands in the air, Paul quietly dying of humiliation. The other carpets came down, the ride stopped and we de-carpeted, though I was not pleased. I was angry.

Paul, ever the optimist, figured that perhaps that particular carpet was just broken, maybe it wasn't us? So we stood around afterward to watch the next round and alas, another family of four was stuck on the bottom turning round and round. There was clearly a broken carpet (though it was inexplicably a different color than ours had been).

I had paid nearly £400 just for entry into this place, and would have saved £140 had I simply come the day before the twins turned 3. I had spent 80% of my time so far that day standing in lines. We waited an hour and a half to see Goofy, just as we walked in the entrance. We lined up for an hour to ride a merry go round for less than a minute. We lined up to use the bathroom, which was so vile and dirty that I'm still considering sending an angry letter to Disney over it. (And I've seen some AWFUL bathrooms in my travels) The line just to get into a restaurant was over an hour. I'd had enough. I had not stood in line for 20 minutes to get onto a broken carpet!

So I did something that Canadians so rarely do abroad –
I complained. To a French speaking Disneyland
employee standing near the exit of the ride. Her English
wasn't great, causing me to descend into the bizarre
traveler's phenomena of "if they don't understand my
language it must be a volume problem", and started
speaking louder and louder until I was nearly shouting.
At Disneyland. In partial French. This drew somewhat
of a crowd.

The woman was still struggling to understand the
language and volume of my issue, so I resorted to
including charades and large, sweeping hand
movements. Paul took the twins by the shoulders and
backed slowly away. A larger crowd formed as I quite
audibly complained that I had waited 20 minutes in line
for a broken carpet and that there are absolutely no
weight limit signs posted, nor did the ride operator raise
any concerns when coming round to check our safety
bar before the ride started. This was unfair, my children
were upset (more so because of me, admittedly) and I
expect someone to put a stop to families from being put
onto a broken carpet-car!

She kindly confirmed that she would "take care of us"
and, pulling us away from the gawking crowd she took
us through to the Fast Pass lane of the ride, with
everyone in the long line watching us walk through to
the front – the same people that had watched us clearly
fat-break the ride a few minutes earlier. Satisfied, but
convinced that the trick was to nab a blue carpet this
time, the girls and I went up to the gate. Paul chose to

leave the girls with me and climb up to a picture point to get a photo of us going around.

The gate opened and I told the girls to run for the blue carpet, go go go! We got it, though the girls sat with me in the back of the car. We were good, hopefully with only one adult in the carpet the thing would go up, right?

Just as the ride was about to start the operator rushed over with one more family – another overweight woman with her young son.

Craaaaaaaap. Crap crap crap crap crap.

After the humiliation. The scene I made with that poor, poor woman. The march of shame to the front of the line. We were doomed to ride around the bottom yet again.

I looked up at Paul as he mouthed "Sorry" from his perch up top.

Just as I considered getting out early and making yet *another* scene, a faint announcement came on over the speaker next to us, first in French and then faintly in English:

"To raise the carpet in the air, use the lever in the front of the carpet. To tilt the carpet up and down, use the lever in the back of the carpet."

Oh. My. God. We hadn't fat-broken the ride. We were just complete idiots.

The ride started to go round and we were still at the bottom. Desperate, I nudged the woman in front of me, motioning to her that she needed to use the lever in front of her to raise the carpet into the air. She declined, waving me off with a smile.

I wasn't having it. I was already in too deep. I gave her a forceful nudge and screamed "push the lever!!!" Push it push it push it!!!!! Startled, the woman pushed the lever (and gave me a very dirty look) and, joy of joys, we lifted into the air to the absolute delight of the girls as we sailed round and round, high in the air and past Paul with a massive grin on my face as I mouthed to him:

"Ha! See! Not too fat!!"

Shamed out of Switzerland

So we were nearing the end of our family camping trip across The Netherlands, Germany, Belgium, Lichtenstein, Austria, Switzerland and France with our Honda CRV, a massive tent and our 3 year old twins. Oh, and Sarc. (it's not like I could do a beach holiday now, right?!) We made it to our campsite in Switzerland right by the lake, absolutely gorgeous. Really friendly people, some elderly French campers came by to chat to us to the point that we were trying to back away to keep setting up our tent before darkness really set in. They were chatting with us for so long that we ended up setting up the tent and blowing up air mattresses in the dark, which was getting really frustrating. I'd had the kids pretty much attached to me like koalas for the last few days and they were tired, hungry and just getting into pretty much EVERYTHING.

Tensions were stirring.

I had to pee? They came with me. They either squeezed into the stall with me and watched, commentating aloud to the rest of the bathroom on my bodily functions, or they stood outside the stall with the instructions "Don't. Touch. ANYTHING!" and me calling out their names like a roll-call every 30 seconds to make sure they were still there. Always until either one of them would tattle on the other and shout "Mummy! She's TOUCHING things!" or someone would set off the hand dryer and they would both descend into terrified screams and two three year olds trying to break down and crawl under the bathroom door to get to me, all while I'm flipping out about them touching the floor of a public bathroom. It was a scene nearly every single time.

Paul, however, would go off to pee in the bathroom by himself. Maybe stop to talk to someone along the way. Take his sweet time. Keep his bodily functions to himself.   Like at the French rest stop in which I resigned to just pee with the door open to make life easier for myself for when the kids came screaming in (as they were keeping watch outside the door) at a rest stop without a single other car there, which ended in me

291

completely flashing an elderly British woman. She watched as I straightened in surprise and peed on my own shoes. (Kids were off running in a field with their dad).

Yes, tensions were stirring.

We needed water for dinner? I went, with the kids. He was still setting up the tent. Off we trekked, in the dark. I needed to get the pillows from the car? They came and helped. I cut bread? They helped by running away with the bread in one direction and the actual table in another.

The tent was up. The table was set up and I had begun to cook an elaborate pasta dinner in the dark, aided only by the Lego-Man flashlight I had wedged under my chin. Some friendly Russians drove up and began setting up their tent – Paul kindly offered them our large camping light to help them see what they were doing, while I, his wife, struggled to cut and butter a baguette with a Lego-Man light.

Tensions had risen up nicely by that point.

Paul needed to put a few things away into the car, a mere ten feet away. I asked if he could take the kids with him, as they were currently fighting about "who could sit their chair closest to mum while she's cooking in the dark" and one had situated herself directly on top of my foot. He said that his hands were full and he couldn't possibly take them.

I threw a chair. The Russians saw.

Taking the hint he took the kids to set up the tent bedding, the Russians brought back our primary light source and we sat down to a nice dinner and a lovely evening of chatting, relaxing and cuddling under the stars. Very nice. Picture perfect family once again, and we went to sleep as usual with Paul and Lochie on one side of the tent and Kaitie and I sharing the other.

Everything was calm until one in the morning that night. Kaitie was too hot and she started kicking off our covers by lying (sleeping) on her back and kicking her legs up into the air and slamming them down repeatedly to get out of the blankets. This woke me up (like a good, attentive mother) and I turned my face to see what she was doing when WHAMMO! Down came her heel directly into my open eye and I screamed "Owwww YeaaaaaaaghhhhHHHHH!!!!!! My Eyyyyyyeeeeeee!!" to which she started crying and screaming. Oh the electric shock of pain that had taken over my eye socket. We were both crying and screaming, with me writhing around on the air mattress trying to right myself in the dark and holding my face in my hands, her bouncing around helplessly with the momentum of the flailing air mattress like a trampoline. She even started to giggle. It was a scream-giggle. Her twin in the other sleeping area with her dad was shouting "I want a turn!", I was yelling to Paul "I'm blind! I'm blind!" to which he responded "It's dark, we all are!"

It must have looked and sounded as though a bear had gotten into the tent. Paul's yelling to see if I'm okay, I'm crying, Kaitie is cry/laughing and Lochie is enraged that her mattress isn't bouncing around like a rodeo bull too. Kaitie actually bounced off the side of the tent and clear to the opposite end of the mattress. It was just some kind of hot mess all around.

In the morning I emerged from the tent with a shiny black eye and both the Russians and the French completely avoided making any kind of eye contact with any of us. The four of us ate our breakfast in silence and exile.

We checked out at noon, a day early, and felt it best to just leave Switzerland all together.

I didn't think a HAZMAT bunker would fit down there

I sometimes think that if I weren't there to witness these things that I would barely believe them myself.

Dr. Sarc looked up at me from over my massive blue medical file – pages bulging out of reinforced clips bearing a lifetime of medical history covering the span of only two years. My condition was raging – eyes red and limbs swollen and stuck out like the Michelen Tire Man. "This is concerning" he said.

It wasn't the first time I'd been branded 'concerning' by a medical doctor, nor my first experience as the

Michelen Tire Man. Upon first arriving in China a full medical was required in order to work as a kindergarten teacher, including (and especially) a test to see if you had any sexually transmitted diseases that could be transferred to the children (my thoughts on the job description of kindergarten teachers do not generally include activities of the nature in which an STD can be transferred to children, but oh well. When in Rome.). Weight vs height must be taken and the hospital was keen to try out its new fancy electronic scale on its very first foreigner, so there was, of course, a crowd. This wonderful scale displayed not only a person's weight but also an associated pictograph of the person's general health – ranging from ill looking stick figure to happy stick figure, going so far (as had been explained to me) as a reasonably plump looking stick person on the high end. The crowd prepared and ready, I stepped onto the scale.

Michelen Tire Man. I kid you not. The staff hadn't even known that picture was an available option. It was *actually* a picture of the Michelen Tire Man. Even had the hat.

Dr. Sarc continued to leaf through my oversized file as I reminisced fondly over my memories of China and good health, Michelen Tire Man or not. "I'd like to get a baseline of where your body is affected by inflammation" he mused. "your children are still quite young, can you stay in a hotel?"

Wait, what?

Sometimes keeping up with a doctor's train of thought is like trying to herd cats. I've recently adopted the 'sure, why not?' approach to my responses, as things tend to work out better if I just go with the flow.

"You've been booked for a Gallium Scan at the end of this week. It is like a CT scan of your full body but with Gamma Radiation that will highlight any active inflammation."

Oh cool, like Bruce Banner!

"Who?"

You know! Gamma Rays. Bruce Banner. The Hulk. Raaaawr!

Silence.

I guess you have to know your audience. My husband and his brother at least thought it was pretty cool – though the technician wouldn't let me take pictures inside the room, nor would she take a photo of me in the machine pretending to get superpowers. You would *think* that a Gamma Ray technician would be a comic book fan. You would think. Seriously.

I was shot up with radioactive 'stuff' (stuff being the most technical word I could remember) and told to stay away from any young children or pregnant women for at least two days, which was difficult as a mother but we got through it. The problem was more so the trip we had booked with my mother in law to drive through

Western Europe starting a couple of days later – too late to get a letter from the hospital confirming the *reason* I was so radioactive should anything go amiss. Ah well, what's the worst that could happen? My husband's visa renewal had been delayed by the Home Office of the United Kingdom so he was travelling on a passport without a visa to return to the UK anyway – we figured being a little radioactive would be the least of our worries and just went with it.

The trip was fantastic – we drove through France, Belgium, The Netherlands, Germany, Switzerland and Lichtenstein before returning to Calais in France to board the ferry back to England – with me wedged in between the twins in the back of our little blue Honda CRV. As Canadians the border controls within Europe surprised us for the little enforcement we experienced, having re-entered France from Switzerland and stopping voluntarily at French Customs, despite no seemingly obvious requirement to do so. I gathered our passports and got out of the car, nervously approaching the bored looking border guard while glancing back at my eagerly watching family for moral support. I was nominated to go as I had the best non-existent French.

I approached the guard with his feet up and poking through the gate cubicle window. I said hello and introduced myself, in French. He didn't care. He didn't really look at me until I tried to thrust five Canadian passports into his hand, asking if we can get stamps and go. He handed them back without looking at them, saying something quickly in French. I didn't catch it. I asked him in English if we could please have our stamps and go, did we need to do anything further? He replied that he didn't speak English. We were stuck. I had our passports and seemingly his permission to get back in my car, but this just seemed wrong. Too easy. Going through customs in Canada and America is like being caught sneaking in drugs by the KGB. A Canadian official once grilled us for ten minutes on the material used for a cheap cardboard puzzle of Stonehenge we had brought back for Paul's family. A Chinese official once gleefully tore through my suitcase pulling out various items such as copious amounts of Tylenol, Pepto Bismol, dental floss and condoms (the kinds of things you bring in bulk when living as a foreigner in China) yelling at the top of his lungs in broken English about " so much Sex and Drugs!" to my extreme public humiliation. A Jamaican Border Guard once dumped my suitcase upside down onto the tarmac looking for drugs and then held his AK47 on me as I hastily packed it back up an ran for the plane. The Thai were a relaxed bunch, surprisingly. So I was very much caught off guard when the French customs official not only wanted nothing to do with us, but seemed to want me to just leave . He called over his sleeping colleague, whose English was supposedly better than his.

They had a very long conversation in French full of gestures, to which the second officer translated back to me as "Just go".

That's it' Just go? Really? It sounded like a whole lot more than that. Are you sure? You don't want to search us or anything? Check Interpol records? Make sure those are really my children?

"Just-e, go".

You're sure. Really? Okay, if you say so…

The first officer then got involved again, sticking his chin high up in the air and motioning with a dismissive flick of his hand – "Just-e, go". They both turned away from me to confirm their disinterest and I scurried back to our car – completely confused by the exchange yet happy to be back on our way and getting the hell out of the weirdness that was Switzerfrance.

The lax customs throughout Europe had given us a false sense of security when it came to re-entering Britain, as upon parking our car in line for the Ferry my husband without a visa was pulled off into a refugee holding area to be questioned by UK Immigration officials while the rest of us were not permitted to leave the confines of our car. He was the sole Canadian sat amongst a mixed group of refugees, caught illegal entrants handcuffed to the wall and sobbing families huddled together. The group took great interest in him, all wanting to know what he was possibly in for and had he been caught inside a truck as well? Oh no, he explained. The Home Office just lost my biometrics and didn't send me a visa in time, so I'm just travelling with a letter of approval that there is some confusion about. But the best of luck with your Asylum application, I'm so sorry for your losses. And… um…. good luck with that.

In the end a border official returned to release my husband from the holding cell with apologies for having detained him and assurances that everything was just fine, they got in touch with the caseworker and his new visa will be put into the post today, you can re-join your family (who were now no longer under car-arrest) and board the ferry, welcome back to the UK.

Shaking our heads and thinking that was the last of the trouble we would experience on our trip we boarded the ferry, relaxed as it crossed the channel and piled back into our car, me again squished between the twins in the back seat, for the drive back to London and the return to life as we knew it. Except we still needed to go through customs, as drivers. Just drive through these big Jurassic Park looking cement gates to be waved through by a vested official and we would be on our way home. Cars were being put through at a slow, regular pace as we drove into line, creeping our way toward the other side of the enormous gates and on to the freedom of being back in the UK.

The line seemed to slow to a crawl once we got in it and closer to the gate of freedom. Bars began to pop up alongside our car and the car behind us was stopped by an official, holding the line back. We continued to creep forward, following the car in front of us until they too were stopped by an official. Once our car was fully stopped red lights lit up all around us and small claw-like contraptions sprang up in front and behind our car, preventing us from driving either forward or backward for fear of ripping off our tires. A customs official in a bullet proof vest appeared, directing us to drive to the right and down into the tunnel that we had just noticed was there, the doorway having slid open to await our vehicle.

Well *this* seemed a bit intense.

We drove down into what looked to be a large cement bunker, large enough to hold about three large semi-trucks and to contain an explosion. No windows or even an office to be seen as the door slid closed behind us and we were left there, five bewildered Canadians huddled inside a blue family CRV in the middle of a large, empty cement bunker. This was one of those things that people talk about seeing just before a government makes them disappear, surely. We didn't dare get out of the car. My husband had been handed a laminated leaflet stating happy and reassuring things in multiple languages like "please be patient as you have been randomly selected for further checks". I didn't know what kind of random checks required a large cement underground secret bunker but hey, not much can surprise me at this point.

About twenty minutes later a UK Border Agency customs official appeared, wearing hazardous materials gear, including a mask. This was a bit alarming. She was holding what looked like a transistor radio and came to my husband's window, explaining to him that their sensors had picked up what seemed to be an alarmingly high level of radiation from within the back of our vehicle consistent with chemical weaponry – were we carrying anything that we wanted to declare now?

It was at this point that my husband burst out laughing (not a reaction she was anticipating) and said "that's not a chemical weapon, that's my wife!"

We hastily explained to her that I had a medical condition and had recently undergone a gallium scan, which involved a large amount of radiation and didn't actually give me any superpowers (how does nobody find this funny?), but I was medically cleared to be around children and pregnant women so we're sure I'm fine.

The woman took a good look at me as I did my best to look sickly, despite having obviously just been coming back from holiday. I offered to get out of the car to talk this through but was denied, none of us were to get out of the car until this was sorted out. She had us roll up the windows as she turned on her Geiger counter thingy and began to slowly walk around the car, pointing it toward us as she did. She started at the front of the car, pointing her little radiation reader toward the hood as it emitted a slow, rhythmic beeping sound. Beep, beep, beep, beep. No major concern so she proceeded to move along the right side of the car, slowly reaching the point at which my husband sat with his hands placed nervously on the steering wheel. She pointed the machine directly at him and the beeps sped up and increased in pitch ever so slightly. None of us said a word during this exchange, not even the twins who were taking their cues from the tension of their parents sat nervously in the car, confident that there were no chemical weapons hidden in the back of the car but unsure of what would happen should they not believe us.

The hazmat clad officer then proceeded along to the middle of the car, where I was sitting with the twins and she jumped back in alarm as the machine's sounds graduated from a slow and rhythmic beep, beep, beep to a high pitched and urgent *beep-beep-beep-beep-beep* with flashing red lights. Even the Geiger counter sounded scared. The woman looked from her machine back to us and resigned herself to keep going around the car, the boot of the car showing nothing of note and the same thing happening again once she got to the other side of me, the machine calming again at my mother in law – who was nearly in tears and on the cusp of a nervous breakdown. (and she had traveled with me previously, she'd even been there for the sobbing plane incident near Hong Kong. I still maintain that the woman knew what she was likely in for when she signed up to travel with me).

The officer returned to my husband's window, reluctant to have any direct interaction with me, and explained to him that this was all very odd, the Geiger counter she had must surely be broken and she would have to get another one. We would need to hold tight.

Another twenty minutes and despite having had a good laugh about it as a family in the car the situation was quickly approaching 'no longer all that funny' as we were anxious to get home or at least see the outside world again.

The officer returned, this time flanked by three senior officers who explained to us that they had had to send out for another machine that was better calibrated, it shouldn't take too long. They were much more friendly with us and chatted, even leaning up against our open windows having been reasonably satisfied that we probably weren't terrorists. Probably. They laughingly explained that everyone 'out back' was shocked to find that we were just a typical family on holiday, as the radiation readings that had come up showed me being 'more radioactive than a truck full of Russian uranium coated nails'. They would *obviously* be concerned. When I asked if it was safe for me to be around my children they only kind of hesitated before responding "probably".

Another half an hour and two more Geiger counters later we were cleared to go, the special 'American' Geiger counter having confirmed my radiation as 'medical gallium'. We found out, through our casual chat with the Hazmat suit clad customs officers while being detained in our car within the cement bunker, that the Americans had apparently sponsored an anti-terrorist effort involving rather expensive equipment being given to 'lesser equipped' target countries like Britain, Australia and Canada for the purposes of detecting and stopping terrorists before they become American problems – of which we were pleased not to have become. I have a hard enough time with my mother in law loving me despite my vegetarianism, I cannot imagine the damage an unplanned trip to Guantanamo Bay would do to our relationship.

We were released and sent on our way with chuckled apologies and jokes about Russian nail toting terrorists, eager to be out of that bunker and back on the free and open roads of the United Kingdom. We were 'home', we were free, we had made it and I leaned back to enjoy the peace and calm that had come over the family as we drove along and entered the motorway.

Not even five minutes of driving on the motorway and enjoying our civil liberties when my husband burst out with "You know how I can tell we're back in the UK? Everyone's driving like they've got brain injuries, that's why!" and "Where do you think *you're* going you creeper!" and then "It's not the Grand Prix, it's just a motorway you muppet!"

Ah. It's good to be home.

Sneaking into China with a bag full of chemo needles and no passport. As you do.

My mother started a fun game on Facebook the other day with her sisters called "where in the world is Candace" and took bets on which currency they would need to send bail money in.

Surprisingly, I'm not a drugged out 19 year old backpacker but a professional, 31 year old married mother of two toddlers. And I still get myself into this type of trouble.

Out of the blue on a Tuesday, a key business meeting opportunity arose in China that I should attend, flights were booked and we were due to leave on Friday. Calls were made to the Chinese embassy in London, favors were called in and my Chinese visa has been arranged for a miraculous one-day service. I made my way down there, everything was submitted and everything seemed good – but it was rejected. My Canadian passport expired in 4 months, not the required minimum of 6 months for any visa to any country, including many countries in which I don't require a visa, but can't get into without those precious 6 months of remaining passport validity. (Like Taiwan, I soon discovered the hard way).

Defeated, I returned to the office and told my boss that I couldn't make it. He wasn't having it. More calls were made. Bigger favors were called in and the embassy had agreed to "view my case outside of the rules for this particular occasion". I returned the next day to the embassy, handed over my passport and again returned to the office. We got a call at 10am. There had been a political dogfight in the embassy and somebody pulled the plug on my visa. We were due to leave tomorrow.

My boss still wasn't having it.

More calls were made, old friends were contacted and it was determined that if I could somehow land in a particular airport in a particular city in China as my first point of entry, I would possibly be given a visa. It's the getting there that would be the problem, as airlines won't let you fly to China without a visa. Apparently if they do, you get deported (and to where, exactly?) and they get a massive fine.

306

So we figured we'd risk it.

Or more so, I'd risk it, and he'd fly directly from London to Shanghai. If I could, the plan was to meet him there by Monday morning. Somehow.

My initial flight was cancelled (British Airways direct from London to Shanghai – it sounded heavenly) and I booked a one way flight from London, through Paris to Seoul, South Korea. There's something rather intimidating about booking a one way flight to a country in Asia that you've never been to and have no intention of staying in for more than a couple of hours with nothing to get you onward or backward but an envelope of cash, a reasonably valid passport and your iPhone. But that's how we roll around here. A further one way flight was booked for me from Seoul to China, but I'd worry about that if and when I got that far.

My problems started in London when they didn't want to let me check in. My passport was okay, they didn't bother counting up the remaining months, but they could see that I had a further flight booked to China and I was lacking in said visa. They didn't want to let me through. I explained that I just had to get to the airport in China and that a visa would be arranged for me. They wanted to see paperwork explaining that, but of course, I had none. I couldn't even give them a named contact that was arranging this because well, this type of thing isn't normally done. Korean Air finally agreed to let me on to the Paris flight, but I would have to pick up my bags there and talk to them again about the next leg.

Once in Paris, the same song and dance ensued.

"You don't have a visa for China"
"Really?"
"Yes, you need a visa for China."
"Oh yes, that. It's all been arranged."
"If it were all arranged, it would be in your passport."
"Excellent point. How about you just check me in to Seoul, then."
"But what will you do when you get to Seoul?"
"Not sure, but I've got an 11 hour flight to think about it."

He was French, what did he care if some pathetic Canadienne got herself stuck in Korea and deported?

So I thanked him and went on my way.

Once I got to Korea things really got interesting.

I was not allowed to check in for the China flight, because I did not have a Chinese visa. They did not buy my spiel of it being pre-arranged without any evidence of such. My word did not seem to count for very much. However, a loophole was discovered – they would transport me to China without a visa *if I was transiting through the Chinese airport directly onto an international flight out of China within 24 hours of landing there and without leaving the airport.* Good enough for me, and off I scrambled to find a travel agency in the airport that could/would sell me a ticket that met such conditions.

After an hour I found a travel agency that could A: sell
tickets internal to China and B: understand that I didn't
need a ticket from Seoul to China, just from China out
and that it had to be within 24 hours of landing. And
couldn't be back to Korea. That left my only options as
Taiwan or Hong Kong, but as the flight to Taiwan was
leaving exactly 23.5 hours after my arrival in Shenyang
and met the strict conditions of the transit visa for the
purposes of Korean Air, I bought it. A non-refundable
one way ticket to Taiwan that I had no intention of
using. Fantastic.

Full of pride at "getting around the system" I
triumphantly marched back to the Korean Air desk and
checked in, explaining that I didn't need a visa because
I was just transiting through, look, here's proof! My
proof was accepted and I was nearly there when – crap
– she noticed that my passport was only valid for 4
months and not the required 6 to get into Taiwan.

Rats. They got me.

I tried explaining that I wasn't actually going to
Taiwan, that this was just a ruse to get into China
(honestly is apparently not always the best policy) and a
manager was called. Fantastic.

I was told that no, they would not take me to China
because I couldn't then get into Taiwan. However, they
agreed to call the manager of the Chinese airport to see
if they would accept me on this type of transit visa, but

it would probably take a lot of time because they are all very busy and I will probably miss my flight anyway, and to go sit down.

That's when I pulled out my final card, and made a call to my boss.

About 10 minutes later he calls me back, tells me what's going on and has me go back to the Korean Air manager. She sees me and says that she's tried, but the line is busy and she hasn't been able to get a hold of anyone there yet. I tell her not to worry, the manager of the airport is going to call her.

She was visibly surprised by this, as were her other two fellow managers and the two check in clerks gathered around them. I returned to my seat in the waiting area and picked up my book again - a couple of minutes later I hear their heels briskly clacking on the floor toward me and look up to see brand new expressions on their faces- they are so very sorry for delaying me, this man is here to take my bags and these two ladies are here to help me check in. Unfortunately, the flight doesn't have a first class area but they have arranged for me to have three seats to myself so that I am as comfortable as possible, and would I like a complimentary lounge pass? Any issue with the bag full of chemo needles and more prescription medication on me than a Columbian drug mule? Not for VIP's, apparently. They can take whatever they want to China – including the two bottles of Jack Daniels' Whiskey I also picked up in Seoul to help me not get arrested once I arrived in China, courtesy of the Korean airport officials for 'their friends in the Chinese airport''.

I'm sure they googled me after I left to see who the in the world I was that I had this much pull in China. I figure that life is short and with being ill it seems even shorter than it did before. Sometimes you have to just wing it and embrace the adventure.

And Shanghai was lovely that time of year.

Ridiculously diseased or not, I still have a vibrant, burning need to live and experience life to its fullest as I can. I have recently been given the 'all clear' from the Stroke Clinic to fly again (I have been grounded for a year now!) and we celebrated by booking a family trip to Norway to see a hip-hop concert. As you do. What is in Norway? No idea. But we're going, we're taking the kids and I'm hoping for at least one good story out of the trip.

Because there is really no point in going, otherwise.

Sarcoi-what-sis?

After months of my doctors trying to get funding approval I was finally authorized for Infliximab treatment as of January 1st, 2014. My doctors called and we started treatment that very week. My cousin and uncle are on this same drug for a different condition – their reviews were glowing. Their advice? Bring a blanket and don't get sick. Okay, that's not too bad, I can do that. The nurses of the infusion clinic, friendly and familiar with me after my 13 months of cyclophosphamide treatment, were excited for me. Infliximab is *the* drug, they said. Patients on Infliximab would come in every couple of weeks like they were filling up at a petrol station. They weren't in the infusion clinic all depressed and scared – they were there for a quick top-up and then on with life.

I was practically drooling with anticipation.

I had my first infusion and felt fantastic, aside from a bit of sudden narcolepsy. For the next few days I felt wonderful and yet surreal. For the first time in a very long time I didn't feel any pain at all. Not a single joint throbbed, not a single bone ached. My eyes felt clearer. My thoughts were clearer. The headache was actually, finally gone. I had energy, and one morning I woke up with the sun shining outside, turned over to my husband and suggested that we go canoe shopping.

As though that was something healthy people did.

A few days later, however, the effects started to wear off. My symptoms returned and I was devastated. I knew that this drug would take a couple of infusions to really take hold, but my hopeful optimism had taken over. I was devastated.

I emailed my doctors a picture of my red eyes and they called me back in for the sarc-clinic later that week, they hadn't quite been expecting this either. At the clinic I saw one of the junior specialists, a brilliant and gentle doctor working under Dr. Sarc. He checked my joints, my red eyes and swollen neck. He felt the heat coming off my cheeks and spots of my limbs. Taking a deep breath, he resigned himself to go bother Dr. Sarc down the hall for an opinion. I wasn't sure about this.

"Oh wait, are you sure we need to bother Dr. Sarc with this? I'm sure it's fine, maybe it will go away on its own?"

Nope. He was pretty sure we needed to consult Dr. Sarc on this one. Mine was a severe case and there was too much risk involved not to check.

"I'm sure he's quite busy though. I have another infusion in four weeks – maybe I should just hold on until then?"

He didn't think I could, and with a final "don't worry, I'll be right back" he left, leaving me sat in his office and panicking about being a bother to the great Dr. Sarc.

Nothing is more alarming than your doctor returning from a 'consult' with the great Dr. Sarc speechless and in a bit of shock. He came in, clutching my giant folder of notes and looking at me with a mix of pity and concern. He quietly and calmly walked into the room to stand in the corner, as though gathering his thoughts before speaking to me. He then said aloud, to no one in particular, "Well I wasn't expecting *that*."

My mind jumped all over the place in an instant and my heart fell. "He said to just leave it be and come back for the next infusion in four weeks, didn't he." It wasn't even a question, I'd started getting to my feet to make a bolt for the door lest I let my disappointment show.

"No, actually, we're going to do both the cyclophosphamide and the Infliximab at the same time."

Wait, what?

I asked him if that was a common approach. He confirmed that no, it wasn't. In fact, he'd not heard of it before and it seemed quite extreme. Safe, but extreme.

Well, safe-ish.

He booked me in for a top-up cyclophosphamide infusion the following day and off I went, leaving him in his bewildered state and going on my way, mind racing. This was another of those things that I had no control over, no point in worrying about it, right? Having no 'real' people to turn to for experience and advice I turned to the online sarc forum, Inspire, asking the people there if they had heard of this approach before. They hadn't. Some wished me luck. Some encouraged a second opinion. Some commented that it had been nice knowing me.

I arrived early at the infusion clinic the next day, the nurses there surprised to see me. What was I there for? they asked. I'd just been there two weeks ago. When I told them about the mix I was met with 'are you sure?' and looks of extreme concern. They hadn't heard of such a mix either, though they figured it was 'probably safe', as long as Dr. Sarc knew about it.

I was feeling confident and relaxed until the infusion ward doctor came up to me, knelt down by my chair and checked that I was 'okay' with this. That kind of raises a red flag, but hey. Dr. Sarc hadn't yet led me astray. I confirmed that yes, whatever he advised I was on board with – my degree is in business, not medicine. Satisfied, but still concerned, she left.

It had been a couple of hours and pharmacy had still not sent up the infusion. The head nurse came to my chair to let me know that pharmacy was taking longer than usual, they weren't happy with the risks associated with mixing the two drugs – but the doctors have assured them that it is alright. Pharmacy is just doing a bit of extra checks now, that's all.

I beat back the giant red flag that had risen in my mind with a baseball bat of denial. It would be fine. This is totally normal, I'm sure this kind of thing happens to

315

everybody. Not a big deal. Plus, it's comforting that everyone is being so thorough.

Right?

Another hour passed and a team of three pharmacists arrived at my chair, looking like models (what is *with* British pharmacists in hospitals? It's like their final year of pharmaceutical studies is held at a Swiss finishing school. I mentioned this once to my husband who was rather matter of fact about it. "There's a drug for everything – they have knowledge and access". I should have been a pharmacist.) and looking down at my bedraggled, hastily ponytailed self with concern. Was that pity I saw in their eyes? They first asked me if I was absolutely certain that I wanted to get this mix of infusions, and had the risks been explained to me? Yes, that I would have pretty much no immune system at all (great!) and was at great risk for infection, blah blah blah. I assured them that it was fine, I'd take certain precautions like getting my heroin from a proper dealer with clean needles instead of 'that guy in the park' and would do my best to refrain from licking the hand rails on the London underground. The Victoria's Secret Models / Pharmacists stared at me, clearly they didn't find my nervous tic of making bad and socially awkward jokes as charming or funny as I did.

Satisfied, they left, to be replaced 45 minutes later by the Head Pharmacist, a stern looking woman holding a very large book. I quickly decided not to crack any bad jokes, no matter how nervous I was, for fear that she would whack me with it. She started off with "Mrs.

Lafleur, I am going to be quite honest with you…"
which is never, ever a good sign. She told me that it
was taking a long time to prepare the drug in the
pharmacy because nobody had dealt with this particular
mix of infusions before and, even though the doctors
are confident with it, the pharmacy is not comfortable
signing off on this. They've had to get someone higher
up to come in to sign off on the whole thing. Am I *sure*
that I want to do this?

I beat down the flaming red flag in my mind with my
baseball bat of denial once again and in a weak voice
assured her again that yes, let's go for it.

A short while later a nurse arrived wheeling over my
infusion tray, the cyclophosphamide bag in its plastic
tray and ready to go. She was ready. I was ready. I was
done living like this. I was done with the pain, the
foggy brain… I wanted my life back – for good this
time. Immune systems are highly overrated anyway.
There were risks, there was a good chance that this
whole thing was going to suck royally and go down in
hospital lore as 'and that's how we figured out that
these two drugs don't mix'. This could go horribly,
horribly wrong. Or it could go really, really well.

"Last chance…" the nurse said to me. "Are you ready?"

Sometimes you have to just close your eyes, take a deep
breath and try.

A life worth living

It has taken me some time to come to terms with what has happened to me. This hasn't been easy, though I do tend to minimize my experiences through humor and the telling of a good story. There were times when my husband and I didn't think that I would be leaving the hospital, and those were hard. There was a time as well when I searched for other people 'like me'. I dove into forums and went out to meet people (remember the support group fiasco?) in an attempt to find someone, anyone, that had my disease to the same severity that I did. I didn't find anyone quite like me for years and once I did I was disappointed to find that even though their disease was like mine, their disposition and experience was not. They were depressed. They had stopped working and were maybe struggling to live on benefits or some form of welfare. Some weren't able to qualify, despite clearly needing the help that our society intends to provide, and were struggling with food banks and just finding ways to sustain themselves. Others shamelessly milked the system for all it was worth. Still nobody was like me.

I felt that something must be wrong with me. That nobody else finds this stuff funny – they find it upsetting, stressful, alarming, depressing… a plethora of adjectives that were clearly 'not funny'. I went through the cycle of grief. I expect to go through it again at some point. But why was I so different? Why do I *always* have to be the one that is different? Was my humor masking an upcoming nervous breakdown?

Should I start locking away sharp tools in the home and padding my bedroom?

I then did what Canadians do not like to admit to doing, and I went to a therapist. Yup, I did. I said it. It's out there. Can't take it back now.

takes a deep breath

It was actually one of the best things I ever did for myself. My doctor suggested it, actually. Gently, but she figured that I might need to talk to someone about everything that was happening to me – this actually was kind of a big deal to go through, apparently. She advised me against going to any form of group therapy – not because I wouldn't benefit from it but more so because I would probably be pretty awful for the other people in the group and she didn't want that on her conscience. Sending someone like me into a woe-is-me support group is a lot like having a group cuddle full of Disney fans and then sending in the guy that killed Bambi's mom. It would just be unwise.

So I went to therapy, and to my surprise I found it immensely helpful. I quickly came to see that humor was my very own coping mechanism and there was nothing wrong with that, it was just... a bit different. And that being 'normal' was highly overrated anyway.

More often than laughing about it and embracing crazy I heard people talk about 'fighting' and being a 'fighter' and 'not letting Sarc win'. In my mind you 'fight' against cancer, the flu, a mugger (well, sometimes), a cold, an injury - against these things you can win. You can certainly lose (think mugger with cancer - double threat!), but it is a battle that will ultimately have a winner and a loser.

To me Sarcoidosis isn't. There are members of the Sarcoidosis forum that have had sarc for 40 years or more. In remission, maybe, probably, not really, never was...

I am finding that as I stop fighting 'against' my sarc - if I instead embrace it as my 'new normal' and a part of myself that does not define me but is still a part of me, that I have been able to move forward more freely.

Yes, I have bad days but I no longer view it as 'sarc' that knocked me down. It's more so that it was too much for me because of sarc - so I need to roll with it. If I am fighting this thing and viewing it as my enemy or a threat to me then I struggle to let things happen as they may - I struggle to let go of the anger associated with being ill and weakened.

Sarcoidosis (shudder. I absolutely loathe that word) is a part of me, and will be for the rest of my life in some way or another. I will never get an 'all clear forever' signal. I will never completely heal. I have scars. But it is not my enemy, it is me.

And it's not all bad, either. I have had some of the funniest moment of my life with this disease. I have met some truly wonderful and amazing people. I have met some bat crap crazy people too (always delightful!)

and I have experienced a warmth and acceptance from strangers that no other experience can provide. I have learned so much about my condition, treatments, the human body and the stunning complexity of it and in turn I have used that knowledge to support and guide people in moments of weakness and fear as I sincerely wish someone could have offered to me when I just started out with this, alone and scared.

Sarcoidosis has taught me true empathy and has blessed me with the opportunity to help others and make a difference in their lives that I never would have imagined. I've had people reach out to me from the online forum Inspire and we've hung out at hospitals, laughing at a not-so-funny condition and just brightening their experience. I've answered desperate texts from people in hospital in the middle of the night and I've even gone with two different people with sarc to their doctor's appointments to help to advocate for them. I've met and made some wonderful friends through this, I've learned to slow down and enjoy what I have in the moment and I've learned to live a life truly worth living - as never before has my time stamp been so obvious.

A young doctor saw my condition for the zebra it was when everyone else was thinking it was a horse. The delighted 'eureka' moment that lit up in his eyes as he huddled over his iPhone in the darkened room in A&E is a moment in my life I will never forget, setting me on a journey that has completely changed my life.

That young doctor saved my life. Absolutely. The best thanks I can give him is to make it a life worth living.

***

With Sincere Gratitude

I have such an intense appreciation for the NHS of the United Kingdom, a truly fantastic system full of wonderful characters riddled with quirkiness and compassion. You'll never hear me knock the NHS (except maybe the food) and I wish I could personally thank each consultant, doctor, nurse, receptionist, secretary, health care aide and even the stab-happy phlebotomists. The imaging technicians and the porters. The maintenance guy that helped me out the cubicle I had locked myself into. The student nurses – stab away you guys! What's the worst that could happen? They're already in the right place if you cause an emergency, right? I say stab away! And just know that for all of you that are yelled at, snarled at, vomited on and bled all over there are also so many more of us that sincerely appreciate everything that you do for us. We're often just too wimpy and scared to tell you.

If you have made it this far then I would like to thank you too. This book has been tough for me to write, as it contains a lot of things that I would prefer to forget – which messes considerably with my chosen mechanism of blind denial. It also, however, contains a lot of things that I don't want to forget. Some great times and very funny moments. It is my sincere hope, more than anything else, that my story has made you laugh –

forgetting your own fears and pain for a moment or two. And that the next time you have an opportunity to laugh and embrace the crazy that you choose to smile at the bit of fun to be had in falling apart.

The Foundation for Sarcoidosis Research (FSR) defines Sarcoidosis as:

What is Sarcoidosis? Sarcoidosis (pronounced SAR-COY-DOE-SIS) is an inflammatory disease that can affect almost any organ in the body. It causes heightened immunity, which means that a person's immune system, which normally protects the body from infection and disease, overreacts, resulting in damage to the body's own tissues. The classic feature of sarcoidosis is the formation of granulomas, microscopic clumps of inflammatory cells that group together (and look like granules, hence the name). When too many of these clumps form in an organ they can interfere with how that organ functions.

What Causes Sarcoidosis? No one knows exactly what causes sarcoidosis, but it is probably due to a combination of factors. Some research suggests that bacteria, viruses or chemicals might trigger the disease. Although such triggers might not bother most people, it is possible that in someone with the right genetic predisposition they provoke the immune system to develop the inflammation associated with sarcoidosis.

What are the Symptoms? Sarcoidosis is a multi-system disorder. Symptoms typically depend on which organ the disease affects. Most often the disease will affect the lungs.

- **General**: About one third of patients will experience non-specific symptoms of fever, fatigue, weight loss, night sweats and an overall feeling of malaise (or ill health).
- **Lungs**: The lungs are affected in more than 90% of patients with sarcoidosis. A cough that does not go away, shortness of breath, particularly with exertion and chest pain occur most frequently with the pulmonary form of the disease.
- **Lymph Nodes**: often they are in the neck, but those under the chin, in the arm pits and in the groin can be affected. The spleen, which is part of the lymphatic system, can also be affected.
- **Heart**: Sarcoidosis can cause the heart to beat weakly resulting in shortness of breath and swelling in the legs. It can also cause palpitations (irregular heartbeat).
- **Brain & Nervous System**: From 5% to 13% of patients have neurologic disease. Symptoms can include headaches, visual problems, weakness or numbness of an arm or leg and facial palsy.
- **Skin**: Painful or red, raised bumps on the legs or arms (called erythema nodosum), discoloration of the nose, cheeks, lips and ears (called lupus pernio)

or small brownish and painless skin patches are symptoms of the cutaneous form of the disease.

- **Bones, Joints & Muscles**: Joint pain occurs in about one-third of patients. Other symptoms include a mass in the muscle, muscle weakness and arthritis in the joints of the ankles, knees, elbows, wrists, hands and feet.

- **Eyes**: Common symptoms include: burning, itching, tearing, pain, red eye, sensitivity to light (photophobia), dryness, seeing black spots (called floaters) and blurred vision. Chronic uveitis (inflammation of the membranes or uvea of the eye) can lead to glaucoma, cataracts and blindness.

- **Sinuses, Nasal Muscosa (lining) & Larynx**: About 5% of patients will have involvement in the sinuses with symptoms that can include sinusitis, hoarseness or shortness of breath.

- **Other Organs**: Rarely, the gastrointestinal tract, reproductive organs, salivary glands and the kidneys are affected.

What is the Treatment for Sarcoidosis? Different treatments will work better for different people, and sometimes more than one drug is used. In some cases, no treatment is needed. But, for some patients, intense treatment is required, especially if organs like the lungs, eyes, heart or central nervous system are affected. Treatment is generally done to control symptoms or to improve the function of organs affected by the disease.

While progress has been made in understanding the symptoms and better diagnosing the disease, little is known about who is susceptible to sarcoidosis and the cause remains unknown. With increased research, discovering the cause, improving treatment and finding a cure may be well within our reach.

www.stopsarcoidosis.org

www.inspire.com/groups/stop-sarcoidosis/ is an excellent international forum for people with Sarcoidosis to lend each other support, information and to occasionally have a good laugh about this whole 'being diseased' thing. You'll find me there as Tofumonkey, and I am forever grateful to my fellow 'sarkies' on Inspire for their support and for the wonderful friends I've made. Truus, Bev, Zoe, Kelly, Betty, Loopy – you guys are my inspiration and keep me laughing, even when things really shouldn't be this funny.

Check out www.sarcoidstar.weebly.com for even more info about Sarc and the support available through similar treatments and conditions.

Above all, keep smiling. Keep laughing. Keep *living*. Whatever condition you may have it may control you, it may change you, but it doesn't have to *define* you.